Praise for *Trust the Wings*

In *Trust the Wings*, Schultze stitches scraps of fragmented lives into a finely-pieced quilt of family, with characters so vivid and endearing they're now sewn into me, too. This is a story few could write, and even fewer with Schultze's artistry. A memorable debut.

—Cheryl Grey Bostrom, award-winning
author of *What the River Keeps*

Trust the Wings folds potent story within potent story, and each sings the same theme: loved ones lost—and found.

—Vinita Hampton Wright, spiritual director,
author of several novels as well as *The Soul Tells
a Story* and *The Art of Spiritual Writing*

Schultze weaves a compelling narrative that resonates with every woman who has ever been overlooked, underestimated, or betrayed by systems stacked against her. Aviana's story is a call to trust our own wings and soar beyond the barriers placed before us. In *Trust the Wings*, Schultze captures the fragile yet unbreakable spirit of women pursuing their dreams against all odds. Aviana's voice stayed with me long after the final page—a testament to courage, renewal, and the quiet power of trusting oneself. I'm truly moved by the depth, strength, and resonance of Aviana's story.

—Martha Kombe, President of Nairobi Youth Advisory Council

An intelligent and worthy novel, Schultze's *Trust the Wings* tells a timely and deeply moving story.

—Hugh Cook, award-winning author of *Heron River*

What happens when our pride is pulled out from under us and we must take on the gritty work that no one else will do? In *Trust the Wings*, Barbara Schultze explores what it means to find our own healing growth not through prestige but through caring for the needy—especially when they are ungrateful, uncooperative, unable to return the favor, and heartbreakingly ill. Beautifully written, *Trust the Wings* is a wise and inspiring story.

—Connie Connally, author of *Fire Music*

Schultze welcomes readers on a heart-expanding journey with Aviana, who must find a way to tell herself the truth. This astute novel invites us to consider where we may need to do this very same thing.

—Cynthia Beach, author of *The Surface of Water* and *Creative Juices for Writers*

In *Trust the Wings*, Schultze accurately depicts the oft-misunderstood work of home care nurses and the struggles of families caring for aging parents. Schultze's deep experience with this challenging environment is evident in this well-written and thought-provoking story.

—Carolyn Flietstra RN BSN, Executive Vice President, Home & Community Services, Holland Home

Trust the Wings

Trust the Wings

a novel

Barbara Schultze

The bird rises against a strong head wind, not only in spite of the wind, but because of it. The opposing forces become a lifting force if faced at the right angle.

L. B. Cowman

Acknowledgments

Trust the Wings is the result of twenty-five years of wishing, hoping, scribbling down ideas and incidents, rewriting, almost tossing away the whole project, and finally blending all the ingredients into this story. So I hope that those who encouraged me in the beginning and along the way will forgive my memory lapses on names and faces from years ago. You know who you are, and I'm grateful.

First, I acknowledge my indebtedness to the hundreds of home care and hospice clients and families who allowed me into their homes over twenty-five years as a home care nurse and seven years as a hospice chaplain. You shared your lives with me. Some of your stories were difficult to tell and heartbreaking to hear. In combining, embellishing, and fictionalizing some of them, I pray I have honored the spirit of all of you.

I thank my colleagues who shared incidents while still maintaining confidentiality, who had my back when I was having "one of those days," and who mourned with me over many inevitable deaths. You all are heroes.

Early in the process, I attended Calvin University's Festival of Faith and Writing and sat under the tutelage of great writers and speakers, including Vinita Hampton Wright, John Updike, Lawrence Dorr, Virginia Stem Owens, Luci Shaw, and Elie Wiesel. The 2009 Breathe Christian Writers Conference, facilitated by Cynthia Beach, introduced me to the gracious writer and teacher Cecil ("Cec") Murphy. And in 2024, as I neared the culmination of those twenty-five years, I spent an intense week at another writers' workshop, Scriptoria, with a gifted cohort of fiction writers— Jolene Witvoet, Chris Meehan, Emma Canup, Capi Cloud Cohen, Ingrid Lochamire, Karl VanDyke, Jonell VanDelft, Grace Miller, Mark VanZanten, and Hugh Cook, who led us and became my general editor.

I regret that I can't pull up the names of my fellow writers from The Well writers group, also facilitated by Ms. Beach, from many years ago. Thank you for reading and critiquing my early efforts when this book had a very different trajectory. I hope that you will find it and recognize your fingerprints on it.

The CALL Writers' Group—Karl VanDyke, Joann Holtrop, Kathleen Waggoner, Abe Vreeke, Michele Wagner, Jane Vander-Haagen, Al Mulder, and Lynne DenBesten—kindly but insistently recommended changes to the "final" manuscript. I thank you for your honest feedback and encouragement.

Thanks to my expert consultants: police officer Felix Purdue on the nuances and ramifications of a DUI/OWI and public indecency; building contractor John Hoekenga on joists, concrete, and linoleum; G. Peter Posthumus on all things LGBTQ in the late 1900s; the Ron and June Daniels family, who invited my husband and me to their daughter's Orthodox Jewish wedding; Don Sjaardema, who courageously shared his experience as a POW; Daniel Salcedo, PhD, and Marijke Velzeboer, PhD, founders of Pueblo to

People and PEOPLink, who gave permission for me to fictionalize their Central American work in the diary sections of this novel; and Rachel Lausch, my Central American guide and former college roommate. All factual errors are mine alone.

I subjected family and friends to reading chapters and finally the entire manuscript. I owe them deep gratitude not only for reading but for their honest critiques and suggestions: Bethany Kim, Natalie Hoekenga, Janet Hoekenga, Erin Mishkin, Quin Schultze, Ruth Vis, Dorothy Seven, and Rachelle Oppenhuizen. We still love each other.

I was blessed with splendid editors and proofers, including Erin Healy, Hugh Cook, Robert Banning, and Elizabeth Banks.

Kristin Goble of PerfecType Typesetting did a wonderful job on interior design.

Matthew Plescher brought his amazing artistry to the cover, graciously incorporating my ideas.

I am eternally grateful to my fifth-grade teacher, Marilyn Himmel, who instilled in me a love of nature, especially of birds and trees, that has enriched my whole life.

Part 1

Chapter 1

The starling burst from the potted yew, startling Aviana as she approached the entrance to Denver's Brown Palace Hotel. It swept beneath her umbrella within inches of her face. She spun around to see that it had landed atop the vintage lamppost behind her. How odd, she thought, to see a starling in the city. She stood beneath it and watched as the bird ruffled its feathers to shake off the last drops of rain, then cocked its head to stare down at her. Staring back, she mimicked the starling's action, releasing the spring of her black umbrella and shaking the raindrops onto the rain-slicked sidewalk. She tested the chilly November air with an outstretched palm and, satisfied, wrapped the tie around the flapping panels of the umbrella. She turned toward the entrance, smoothed her dress, and paused to admire the pair of winged dragons in the stained glass above the doorway, before ascending the three steps to the entrance. Behind her, the starling's wings riffled in anticipation.

The hotel's sliding doors whispered apart and Aviana passed between them into the vestibule. The starling, misjudging its timing, crashed into the glass and dropped, stunned, to the pavement.

Startled, Aviana glanced back at the sound and saw the doorman hurrying to remove a limp form.

That's the trouble with all this glass, she thought. It confuses the birds. The pigeons seem to have learned how to avoid it, but starlings are used to wide-open spaces. She sighed and continued through the second set of doors into the spacious atrium.

Immediately she was aware that a couple at the reception desk had turned and had begun to size her up. She reached a hand up to smooth her thick black hair behind her shoulder. Why were they staring at her? Did they think *she* had banged into the glass door? They must think her clumsy when all she hoped to project was poise and confidence. The concierge, too, was looking at her. She glared at him through black-rimmed glasses. He raised a hand toward her as if to offer assistance, and she turned away.

She held herself stiffly—shoulders back, elbows cocked, chin lifted toward the balcony as her eyes swept the room. Was the pianist at the grand piano staring as well? She felt exposed, her black sheath that had seemed so sophisticated—could he detect that it was polyester? And her earrings and drop pendant necklace that had looked fabulous against the black velvet box at the jeweler's— were they obvious to others as cubic zirconia rather than diamonds? What had she been thinking when she decided the bolero jacket spattered with rhinestones was a perfect addition?

She took in a shaky breath, scanning the atrium, then another, deeper breath and stepped out on muscular legs that carried her across the polished floor, conscious of the condescending eyes that might be following her.

But the eyes of another man, standing uncomfortably in the doorway of the Palace Arms Restaurant across the atrium, fastened on Aviana. The tension in his face relaxed, and he broke into a warm smile as she approached. He straightened his tie and stepped forward to meet her.

"Avy! You look amazing." His hand reached out and, without hesitation, she slipped hers into it.

"You're just not used to seeing me without jeans and a backpack, Brad."

"That's true, but my compliment holds. You clean up well!" He drew her in and tucked her arm into his.

Eyes sparkling, she melded into his side. It had been years since she had felt comfortable in a man's presence. She found herself finally trusting in this new relationship. The couple followed the hostess across the plush carpet of the dimly lit dining room, gliding in step, side by side.

The burnished wood paneling and furniture of the room were set off by brass fittings and what appeared to Aviana to be a gold leaf ceiling. Military prints covered the antique silk wallpaper. They passed under a blossoming of French military flags stemming from a central brass pole and approached a private table. The hostess invited them to sit on the burgundy leather banquettes facing each other before a floor-to-ceiling mirror, flanked by tall filigreed brass gates that might have been at home at Napoleon's Château de Fontainebleau.

Brad leaned toward Avy over the white linen tablecloth and whispered, "This place is a far cry from the Denver Diner where we last ate. Are you just trying to one-up me or is this some special occasion I'm unaware of?"

She held an index finger in the air and broke into a coy smile as the server approached with two flutes on a tray and a chilled bottle of champagne. He set the tray on a nearby stand, nodded at Aviana, and placed the glasses before them. He held the bottle by the base, tipped it and let the effervescent liquid slide into the narrow rim of each flute.

She nodded a silent thanks at the server and turned back to Brad. "This *is* a special occasion—to mark the fulfillment of my long-term plan. It's taken years of effort to reach my ten-year goal, but in just"—she glanced at her watch—"fourteen hours I will have made it!" She lifted her champagne and paused. "I didn't expect to have anyone to enjoy it with, but since we've been together I wanted to celebrate my triumph with *you*, you lucky man."

"Whatever it is, you deserve it." He clinked his glass against hers.

Avy had met Brad in graduate school, where they were in the same Master of Health Care Administration program, though she was a semester ahead. She'd been assigned as his peer mentor in his first semester. Then as colleagues, they began sharing insights about their work and eventually started seeing each other outside of class. Avy welcomed his invitation to advance their relationship from platonic to romantic, but she'd only recently felt confident enough in their relationship to hint at her career plans. She didn't want to jinx the opportunity that awaited her. She set down her glass and took a deep breath.

"You know that I'm the nurse manager of the ICU at Saint Stephen's," she said, "but I've been in talks with the board for the past few weeks and everything's moving forward smoothly for an advancement." Her exuberance bubbled out in a birdlike twitter, mirroring the effervescence of the champagne. She returned the flute to her lips and sipped theatrically, lifting her pinky finger toward the gilded ceiling. Brad tipped his glass toward her and lifted it to his lips. "At our meeting tomorrow morning, I know they'll finally offer me that big promotion I've been working toward—chief nursing officer."

Brad swallowed and produced a small, repeated cough. "Sorry," he said, "the bubbles." He cleared his throat and announced, "Well, that news deserves a celebratory dinner in a special place like this. Let's live it up—my treat." He picked up the menu. She followed his lead, but responded, "I can't accept your treat for dinner, since I'm the one who invited you, and our rule's always been that the one who invites pays. So, it's *my* treat."

Brad's palms rose up in submission. "Okay. You win."

"Besides, I want to have the deviled eggs with caviar appetizer. I've read that it's a must have, and I've never had anything as exotic as caviar. I wouldn't think of ordering it if you were paying."

Chapter 2

Avy assessed her image in the reflective surface of the hospital's elevator as it rose silently to the top floor. She had taken more care than usual this morning with her appearance. Normally it made no sense to fuss since masks and hair coverings were required to enter any room in the intensive care unit, but today was different. The elevator passed the second floor, where she ran the ICU.

This morning, her hair, thick and fluid like the cup of strong black coffee on her bathroom countertop, was brushed back from her broad forehead. Deftly, she'd twisted it into a thick plait, tethering it between her shoulder blades. She'd scoured her face rosy with apricot scrub. Religious moisturizing had kept her skin as soft as when she had moved ten years ago from the humid Midwest to the mountains of Colorado, but at age twenty-eight, two narrow crevices already bracketed the corners of her mouth like parentheses. Nascent crow's feet crept from her myopic eyes, suggesting the kind of determination required to climb to the top of an organization. She regretted that her eyes, still her best feature she thought, hid behind glasses, but the dry air of the medical center made it impossible to tolerate contact lenses.

Now, rechecking her reflection in the elevator, Avy touched up her lips with her favorite lipstick—Drumbeat Red—to match her blouse, and smiled in satisfaction. She was ready. The elevator purred to a stop at the sixth floor. The mirrored doors slid open, and she strode out on raven-colored heels in her dove-gray, pencil-skirted suit.

This was the day that all her hard work would pay off. The year 2000, with its timely arrival in just two months, would be a milestone in her career as much as it was a milestone for the rest of the world. Her ten-year goal was within her grasp. She had given Saint Stephen's eight years of loyalty and taken every opportunity to increase her education and advance to this point. Her MA would be awarded next month and she pictured the framed certificate hanging on the wall of her new office beside her other accolades that were gathering dust on a closet shelf.

Her dinner last night with Brad had opened a window into the kind of circles she would be mixing in after today. Just recalling his dark chocolate eyes melting in both respect and desire left a satisfied smile on her face, and a blush on her cheeks. She banished that tantalizing memory as she reached the end of the hallway.

She pushed open the glass door leading to the executive suite with a sense of entitlement. This was her world now. The diminutive secretary nodded, affirming that she was the expected Aviana Lehrer, and ushered her to the boardroom door. Conversation tapered off as, alight with anticipation of their welcome and congratulations, she entered the room. The five gentlemen within—she recognized the board members and the president from her previous interview—stood as the door shut silently behind her.

"Aviana, thank you for coming." The president offered his hand, then indicated a seat for her at the far end of the dark walnut table. The other four suits murmured welcomes as she made her way to the empty chair.

She pivoted to take her seat and noticed there were fewer board members present this time. The woman with the blond Jamie Lee Curtis cut, who had responded with sparkling eyes to her answers at their last interview, was missing. Avy regretted that the woman wouldn't be there to offer congratulations when she accepted the forthcoming offer. But there would be other opportunities in the future to reconnect.

She sat in unison with the others, reveling in the way the upholstered seat gave slightly, conforming to her body's pressure, yet allowing her the firm support needed to maintain a regal posture. She made eye contact with the others at the table, greeting each by the names she had memorized, and bestowed a confident smile on the president at the far end of the table. He returned her smile with a businesslike one of his own. Sunlight poured through the glass wall, bathing Avy in its warmth; she knew that this was where she belonged.

"We want to express again our gratitude for meeting with us over the past three weeks as we sought to find the best candidate for this responsible position," the president began.

"It's been my pleasure."

"Thank you, Aviana. We found your qualifications to be excellent, and your service to Saint Stephen's is exemplary."

Her pulse remained steady and her breathing calm as she waited impatiently for his next words—congratulations and their offer of the coveted position. But she maintained her confident smile and eye contact as he went on.

"However, we have decided to offer the position to another candidate."

Across the expanse of the conference table, his mouth continued to move, but his words were smothered under a low chirr buf-
feting her eardrums, building like a swarm of locusts. The warmth
of the room turned chill, as if the blood in her veins had turned to
winter slush.

Like a whisper taunting her from far away, a name entered
her ears from the still moving mouth of the board president—the
name of the chosen candidate—Brad Montgomery. The blood that
had beat confidently like a metronome through her chest moments
ago became erratic. Her breath stuck in her throat, never reaching
her lungs. Her hands trembled until she pressed them down, gripping the arms of the conference chair.

The president's mouth stopped moving and hung open as Avy
pushed herself up from the chair and stood on nerveless legs. She
noted a thin string of saliva suspended between his lips just before
he snapped them shut. As the others surrounding the table froze
in their seats, he rose abruptly from his chair to intercept her as
she reached the door. He could still look down on her, even in
her heels, and she turned away in disgust from the hairs sprouting
from his nostrils. She pushed past his manicured hand. She must
have spoken, she thought later, but she hoped she hadn't allowed
the words tumbling around in her head to find their way through
her tight lips.

Avy found herself back in the elevator, staring at her reflection,
her eyes glinting above her ridiculously red lipstick. She passed the
ICU on the second floor as she descended to the parking garage.

"Bull thistle!" The epithet echoed in the cavernous space as
the elevator door slid open. Only someone with an unimaginative
vocabulary would have used the crude epithets she had held back
moments before, at least she *hoped* she hadn't uttered them out loud.
Years ago, her mother had taught her alternative words—names

of invasive plant species—to replace the foul language she'd been assimilating from schoolmates, and she had added more to her lexicon of expletives after moving to Denver. She sent a few more well-chosen ones into the empty air with each stride. "Spurge! Chicory! Goatsbeard! Motherwort!"

Avy stormed on clacking heels down the dimly lit ramp, but her formfitting skirt threw off her stride and her ankle turned under her. She caromed off the bumper of a mud-caked pickup and dropped on hands and knees. Gasping in pain and frustration, she crouched like a kicked dog. A trickle of blood inched from beneath her rent stocking down the grimy cement incline.

Humiliation and betrayal washed over her, entering her nose and mouth and flushing down into the trough of her stomach. Sloshing about in the acid there, it gained buoyancy and returned the way it had come. Cold sweat broke out on her forehead, and she heaved onto the bloodied cement. Depleted of thought and volition, she backed on hands and knees against the tire of the pickup just as a car turned onto the slope behind her. Headlight beams glanced past as she crouched there, shuddering.

Her head swam with the unexpected torrent of emotions. How could Brad have used her like this? She should never have let down her guard and allowed herself to trust him.

"That stemsucker!" she screamed. "Stemsucker" fit that bloodsucking fraud perfectly. She could see it now. Like the parasitic stemsucker plant of the Colorado desert, Brad had camouflaged his true nature, hiding it beneath the surface until he had the perfect opportunity to invade her space, leeching all of her work and lifeblood from her, then popping out like a little pustule to steal what should have been hers.

Avy had collaborated with him as a trusted colleague in her master's program, shared her research, and even let him coauthor

a chapter in her thesis. She had let herself trust him, and their col-
laboration had led to what seemed to be mutual attraction. But it
was all a sham. He had familiarized himself with her research and
had used her to build and tailor his résumé to the job description
she'd been working toward for years.

"Thurber's stemsucker! If I ever see his face again—ugh!"

Avy wrenched off her toe-binding heels and gingerly palpated
her right ankle. It was tender, but she needed it to bear weight. She
had to get away from this place.

She hoisted her bruised body up on the truck's fender and
steadied herself before tentatively shifting weight onto her right
foot. She winced and took a few more uneven steps, avoiding the
patch of blood and vomit. Using the parked cars for support, she
limped the rest of the way to her worn red '87 Ford Thunderbird.
She eased gratefully onto the bucket seat, drew her legs in after
her, and pulled the door shut on its creaking hinges. She sank back
and felt her body shaking with anger and humiliation. Then she let
herself sob in the dark, consoling womb of her old car.

———— ◆ ————

Avy had joined Saint Stephen's Medical Center in Denver fresh
out of nursing school. As a new member of the laparoscopic surgery team, she had quickly adjusted to the many hands, demands,
and personalities involved in a busy operating department before
transferring in a few years to the intensive care unit. She liked the
opportunity to use her medical skills in critical care, without having to interact as much with people, since many were comatose or
too sick to make conversation.

Over the years, she had proceeded according to plan to positions of greater responsibility and authority to become the nurse

manager of the ICU. When her doctors were happy and the nurses and techs worked efficiently, she was satisfied. The doctors respected her accuracy and efficiency, and if that meant that the nursing staff excluded her from their gossip and after-hours barhopping, so be it. She wasn't there for the friendship.

Saint Stephen's had been good to her, rewarding her for her dedication and professionalism. And she, in turn, had given them her loyalty. Until today.

But while the offense lay mostly with Brad, his deception was aided by the male-dominated board. They had caved to the patriarchy in the executive suite. They had turned a blind eye to the proven leadership they had enthused about three weeks earlier—her high satisfaction scores, glowing recommendations, promotions, and years of loyal service. Then they'd chosen an unproven male outsider to join the suits at the top. He had fooled them too.

She wondered if that was why the pixie-haired woman had not shown up that morning. She had implied that Avy had the job locked up.

The loyalty she had given to Saint Stephen's swung back in that moment to where it belonged—to herself. She would go where she was appreciated, she decided, where her skills and dedication were acknowledged. She would leave Saint Stephen's and find a place that valued and rewarded her.

She positioned her left foot awkwardly on the gas pedal and turned the key—and nothing happened. She pumped the gas once, twice, and tried the ignition again. Her temperamental Thunderbird remained stubbornly silent in its parking space.

The red car she'd bought used in 1989 at age eighteen had fueled her departure from her father's home and carried her across America's flat plains into the foothills of the Rockies. But it had long since lost its gloss. The odometer read 176,384 miles. And it was prone to quit at the most inopportune times.

Like now.

Avy found the business card rubber-banded to the worn owner's manual, wrenched her flip phone from her leather briefcase, and called the repair shop to have it towed once again.

"We told you last time, Miss Lehrer, that it wasn't worth trying to keep it running."

"But I have to get it fixed. I'm planning to travel."

"Look, I can't take your money anymore. If I even managed to get it running again, it would only leave you high and dry somewhere. I'm willing to tow it in and give you something for parts if you want. At least you're at the hospital where a friend can give you a ride home."

She had no friends, and even if she did, there was no way she would go back in there. Furious, she snatched her briefcase and struggled back out of the car. Indignant at this additional betrayal, she slammed the door and abandoned the car in the employee lot. She hobbled down the exit ramp into the glaring Denver sun, shielding her eyes to look for a cab. Nothing. But two blocks away she spied an auto dealer—Grant's Ford.

Avy took in a jagged breath of the cool air in the dealership showroom. She held it for a moment, then slowly blew it out between shaking lips. Her ankle throbbed. She leaned one arm against the metallic surface of a midnight blue hatchback and lifted the weight off her right foot. Her reflection in the car's finish mocked her. Her carefully made-up face was smudged with mascara beneath her eyes, and strands of hair that had pulled loose from her braid caught in the hinge of her glasses. Her forehead creased with pain and anger, but she straightened and aimed for a chair in the waiting area. Sitting there to catch her breath and to force her mind to plan, she absorbed bits of a song repeating on the speaker:

"Never let it force you down . . . your way . . . move ahead into tomorrow . . . follow what's inside you and do what you gotta do. Never let it force you down . . . do what you gotta do."

She glanced up at the TV screen running ads for the latest model Ford had just come out with. "The New Ford Focus— Expect More" stood out on the screen. She found herself nodding in rhythm to the music and in agreement with the lyrics.

It was time to put this disaster behind her and focus on what was next. A new focus would give her the strength she needed to "move ahead into tomorrow," like the song promised.

Her face broke into a wry grin when she put together her need with the name of the car—a new Focus!

Another ad took over, with a song she recognized—"You Gotta Be"—Des'ree, the British pop star, advising "you gotta be bad, you gotta be bold, you gotta be wiser, you gotta be hard, you gotta be tough, you gotta be stronger, you gotta be cool, you gotta be calm, you gotta stay together."

She was all of those things. She could do this! On the TV, a woman pushed up from a despondent posture leaning against a window frame, lifted her shoulders, and left her empty apartment to drive away smiling in a new Ford Focus.

Avy lifted her shoulders, loosened the hair from the hinge of her glasses, and wiped the smeared mascara from beneath her eyes. As a saleswoman approached, she smoothed her skirt and stood. The woman tactfully ignored Avy's bloody knee poking through the torn stocking. She held out her hand and Avy grasped it eagerly.

"Are you looking for a new ride? I noticed you checking out that sexy little Focus a few minutes ago."

"Yes. My ancient T-Bird has finally succumbed to an inevitable death, but I've decided not to waste time in grief. I'm ready to give it a proper send-off to the scrap heap, and I think I've decided on a new Focus. What can you tell me about that one?" Her chin swiveled to the left to indicate the sleek little hatchback she'd leaned on. She had been in a different mood on her way in, and the car had supported her then. She took it as a sign that it could support her moving forward.

"That one was a special order, so it's got some added features, but the buyer changed his mind once he realized the road clearance might not work for what he wanted. He planned to take it camping in some off-the-grid places so he had us add a splash shield under the engine and skid plates to protect the essential parts of the underbody, like the engine and transmission, the steering linkage, front suspension, gas tank, and the differential. It's not quite tank-grade, but pretty darn close. It's also a manual transmission. Can you drive stick?"

"Oh, yeah." Avy responded with a firm nod of her head and lips puckered into a cheeky grin.

Ninety minutes later, the saleswoman waved goodbye, check in hand for the deposit, and Avy drove away in the hatchback she had leaned on for support on her way in, shielded by its metallic midnight blue exterior. Though her ankle still ached, she managed the gas pedal with her throbbing right foot and controlled the manual transmission with the confidence she had gained learning to drive stick in her high school boyfriend's car.

The next morning, the old T-Bird had already been towed away and she pulled her new car into the empty spot. Avy gave its shiny surface an affectionate pat and, ignoring the ache in her Ace-wrapped ankle, strode up the ramp to the elevator.

When she arrived back on the ICU, her steps matched the rhythm of the song in her head—"You Gotta Be." She resumed control of her unit with a satisfied smile. Her resignation letter, giving them two weeks' notice, waited for the HR director to find when he showed up in an hour, and she had a phone interview lined up for her lunch break.

Chapter 3

Avy had already driven nonstop that morning for five hours when she was alerted by a clamorous screech, warning that her new car was in serious trouble. A memory of the Conoco station she had passed a few miles back flitted through her brain and she regretted not stopping. There was still an eighth of a tank of gas, but maybe she had pushed her new car too far with only two weeks' worth of city driving before she left Denver in the cold dark of the early morning. In the middle of Nebraska, she had been lulled by the flat, empty road ahead of her and had been pushing it well over the speed limit. Now, with no help in sight, she pulled onto the shoulder. She turned off the ignition, but the sound continued. If anything, it grew worse. Every gear seemed to be screaming at her. She leapt out onto the shoulder in a panic.

A shadow passed over her and she raised her eyes. A vast cloud of huge birds flying in massed formation cleaved the sky. As they beat their wings in unison, unholy squawks burst from their throats, reverberating from one to the next as the flock passed above her. They disappeared over the horizon and a hush descended. Stunned, Avy fell back against the fender of her innocently silent car.

"What was that?" One distant squawk answered, as a gray sedan appeared around the bend she had just driven through. It slowed, trailing dust, and pulled to a stop beside her.

"Are you okay? Do you need help?" the frazzled young woman called out the half-open passenger window. Avy could see a surly toddler leaning forward from his car seat in the back, staring at her as if she were an interloper in his self-centered world. She fought to keep her face pleasant, though she had the unnatural urge to stick out her tongue at the boy. She pulled her eyes back to the driver instead.

"I thought my car was dying, but the awful noise was coming from"—she swept her arm up toward the empty sky.

"—the sandhill cranes! You're lucky you got to see them—I mean, if you like that sort of thing. This is about the end of their migration back south. You ought'a be around in the spring when they gather here at the river to go north. Thousands of 'em! It's a real attraction for bird-watchers! Crazy people come flocking in, just like the cranes, from all over the place. To me, you seen one crane, you've seen 'em all. But to each his own. Hey!" She whipped around to the backseat to warn her toddler to stop whatever he was up to. "Gotta go! As long as you're okay," she called, and waved goodbye as she took off up the highway. The boy's eyes followed Avy until she was in his blind spot. Her mouth lifted into a half smile as she waggled her fingers after the car.

Two more cranes winged overhead from the north, burbling in intimate conversation with each other. Their prehistoric appearance was oddly graceful—gray silhouettes sailing across a blue-gray sky, wings beating in rhythm to lift them higher, spindly legs trailing like impractical appendages. Avy felt her heart soar with a primordial yearning to fly free, to join them, but they disappeared south beyond a tree line, and she was stuck on the ground, traveling east.

She shook her head and climbed back into her Focus. She shut the door, stared at the key still in the ignition and took a deep breath. Holding it, she grasped the key between her thumb and middle finger and twisted. The car came to life without complaint, and Avy exhaled in relief. She inched the car off the shoulder and slowly picked up speed. A few miles later, she pulled into a service station to use the restroom and fill the car up. Then, to fill herself up, she bought a twenty-ounce coffee and a sesame seed bagel.

"Twenty-one hours to go to get to Albany if I can keep it to only another couple of stops for gas. Maybe twenty-two realistically." She glanced in the rearview. The Rockies had disappeared. "Catskills, here I come."

Chapter 4

Obsidian eyes in a pale white face appeared suspended in her headlights for an instant before rising past her vision. Screaming, Avy ducked and threw her hands over her face. The car swerved to the right before she slapped them back onto the steering wheel and wrestled for control. She smashed her foot down on the brake pedal as the car slewed onto an exit ramp. With a hope-plummeting squeal, the Focus jolted to a stop on the brink of the exit's central embankment and thunked into silence. The scent of scorched metal rose through the air vent like a noxious wraith. She looked in the rearview and saw a worrisome puff of white smoke painting the dark night.

"Smoke and mirrors and illusions! My brain is in the hands of a magician! Did I fall asleep and dream that disembodied face? Was I hallucinating?" She was too tired to unscramble the illusion right then.

Disoriented, she tried to piece together what had brought her to this precipice. Her brain's neurons, wakened from torpor, fired crazily.

The betrayal by Brad. He'd become a close friend and colleague, and she'd begun to love and trust him. The loss of her hope for advancement at Saint Stephen's. The death of her beloved old car spurring a determination to change her focus—to be bold but cool, wise but tough. To adjust her career plan to a new location far away from the disappointments of the past few weeks. To find a place where she was appreciated and valued.

Her Denver life was hours behind her, and she still had hours to go to reach Albany for the follow-up, in-person interview at Saint Catherine's in three days. If she could get back on the road.

She had no idea where she was.

She had been driving for hours on Route 80, paying no attention to the monotonous voice of the GPS since Route 80 merged with Route 90, and Route 90 would take her straight into Albany. But if the GPS was correct, she was now, inexplicably, on Interstate 94, in her home state of Michigan instead of where she was supposed to be—still driving through Indiana—at least, she was before she swerved onto the ramp. Somehow, she had lost her way while on her way.

Falling snow clouded her vision, but the halogen lights from the Speedway truck stop across the median burned brightly enough for her to make out a tire-sized ring wheeling lopsidedly from beneath her car. "No!" she cried. "Not a wheel!" It rolled down the bank and came to a stop in the snow below. She strained to see down the embankment where it had disappeared, beseeching the car itself to still be intact after all. She breathed in ragged, shallow breaths, loosened her hands from the steering wheel, and stared into the lights of the console. The dashboard clock read 12:17 a.m. She calculated she'd left Denver around eighteen hours ago.

She berated herself. She should've stopped to sleep a while back. But if she stopped, she feared her brain would just remind her, over and over as it had the past two weeks, that she was a fool. She had to put that behind her. She was strong, smart, wise and capable, but she acknowledged that it was a mistake to try to drive across the country in one stretch. She should have stopped in Chicago, she conceded. She could have seen her brother. So, she decided, if she could get back on the road, she'd find a place to crash for a few hours.

She pulled the flashlight from the glove compartment and switched it on. She cracked open the car door and peered into the darkness. The ground appeared nearly a foot farther below her than it should have been. She slid, trembling, from the car and the dormant pain in her upper spine spasmed to life as her left foot dropped onto the loose stones of the shoulder. She steadied herself on the sloping edge, then crouched down in the gravel and shined the flashlight beam beneath the car. All four wheels were still present, but the front left tire was still rotating slowly a foot above the ground and the rear tire was only inches from the shoulder's edge. Thankfully, she saw that the passenger side tires appeared to remain on the asphalt.

She trained the light on the rest of the undercarriage. The front axle balanced precariously atop two steel poles attached perpendicularly by a four-way pipe fitting. Painted white, the whole structure appeared to be a large cross. The once-vertical pole disappeared into a cement-filled oil drum, now leaning sideways out of the earth. So maybe the ring that rolled down the hill was a wreath, she surmised. Beyond the obvious gouges channeled into the skid plates, she couldn't tell if there was any significant damage to the car's vital organs. "Thank God and that disinclined off-roader for those skid plates!" She rose cautiously and brushed the bits of stone and sand from her hands and the knees of her jeans. The front wheel on the driver's side had stopped, while the passenger tire barely held to the asphalt on the right.

An eighteen-wheeler hummed down the highway below and passed out of sight beneath the overpass. The service station across the highway, though lit up like an operating suite, appeared uninhabited. She was alone. She would have to try to get the car back on the road by herself.

It was too cold to remain outside without her coat. Goosebumps already rose on her exposed skin. Anyway, there was nothing she could do from the outside. But getting back inside that precariously balanced car? Entering on the passenger side would be safer, but eventually she would have to get in the driver's seat in order to manage both the clutch and the gas.

On tiptoes, she slipped one hip gingerly onto the driver's seat, imagining her body as weightless so as not to disturb the delicate balance beneath it. The other foot lifted slowly off the ground and settled on the car mat. She eased the door in to graze the frame without catching the lock and leaned her upper body as far as she could into the passenger seat to add weight to that side. The car's underbody complained but held steady.

November snowflakes danced in her headlights and gathered on the windshield. Avy gripped the steering wheel with her left hand, then inched the right one toward the gear shift. She suspended her breathing, depressed the clutch pedal, and coaxed the gear shift from drive, where it had shut down, into neutral. She turned the key and the engine thrummed to life. Her released breath became visible in the cold night air. Before she dared trying to back up, she flipped on the intermittent wipers to clear the flakes from the windshield so she could see—and gasped as a tuft of brown striated feather swept back and forth on the metal arm until the wind snatched it away.

She hadn't been hallucinating! That disembodied white face must have been an owl, she realized.

She inhaled deeply into her diaphragm and slowed her breathing to the steady cadence of the wipers. Disregarding the sounds rising from the underbelly of the car, she turned the wheel, praying the tires would line up with the pavement behind her. She stared into the rearview, shifted into reverse, and gunned the engine. The tires on the passenger side threw gravel into the air, but the car sprang free and rebounded onto solid ground. Avy exhaled in relief and inhaled with renewed determination. As she pulled forward up the ramp, her headlights swung away from a shadowy figure just topping the hill.

"Recalculating."

The bossy GPS voice was still there. Since she exited Colorado, it had been her annoying companion. Across the Nebraska plains, into the rolling hills of Iowa, the stubbled fields of Illinois, and the industrial sprawl of northern Indiana, it kept her moving east on Interstate 80. But at some point in that dark night, she had tuned out the voice and lost her way. Drifting north, she had entered Michigan.

"Recalculating. Return to the highlighted route. Continue straight onto the entrance ramp for Interstate 94 east. Recalculating. Recalculating."

"Chicory!"

She idled at the top of the ramp. Taking 94 east would still bring her into New York on only a slightly longer route. She was awake now, thanks to adrenaline, but it would soon wear off. She realized she couldn't continue like this, exhausted and shaking. She needed to sleep. She punched off the GPS, then turned left. Over the highway, away from the highlighted route, onto Route 131— the familiar road leading north toward her hometown and her father's house—leaving the lights of the Speedway station behind.

An hour later, she approached Berndtbridge on the two-lane rural route. Glaring street lamps lit the concrete span over the river. A hundred yards to the west, the historic covered bridge that gave the town its name still stood. Known as Berndt's Bridge, it straddled the river in semidarkness, illuminated only by tiny white Christmas lights that reflected like stars in the tranquil river below. Closed to traffic now, it was crossed only by bikers and walkers, and anchored the park that had grown up around it.

She decelerated a few minutes later and turned onto Comber Row, the familiar street on the southeast edge of town, then slowed to a crawl in front of a two-story ranch. The yellowed carriage light over the garage illuminated the still-falling snowflakes against the gray siding of the house. The last time she'd seen it, the house wore olive drab. She stopped just short of the driveway, killed the engine, and melted back into the seat.

She began to regret her decision to return to her father's house, where she knew she was uninvited and unwelcome. She should have just found a hotel for the night. She blew out a resigned sigh.

But she was here now. She could just crash on the couch for a few hours so she wouldn't fall asleep at the wheel—again. Then she'd be out of there and on her way. Assuming her father didn't throw her out first when he discovered her there. Yeah, she thought, it was a big assumption.

Avy found the door unlocked, as it had always been, and slipped inside. She let her eyes adjust to the dimness and noted the familiar hollow ticktocking of the kitchen clock that she'd forgotten for ten years, the fusty odor of neglected housecleaning gathered behind window shades that were never opened, and a faint light coming from the top of the stairway, like moonlight pooling on the landing.

Suddenly the quiet was broken by the sound of urgent scrabbling overhead. The fox terrier burst out of an upstairs bedroom and launched himself down the stairs. He threw himself at her thighs, knocking her back against the door. As she slid laughing to the floor, he scrambled over her full bladder and barked desperately at the edge of the door behind her shoulder. She clambered to her knees to reach the doorknob and let him outside to pee in the pachysandra by the entrance. Then she found her own way in the dark to the bathroom tucked beside the basement stairs.

Alex was the bane of her father's life. "Beast of the field," he called the feisty fur-ball. The dog barked at anything that moved, chewed the furniture, and indiscriminately ingested any food within reach of his three-foot leap. He had even learned how to open the screen door and disappear for hours into the nearby woods, returning filthy only at dinnertime. After raising two daughters, producing a son and teaching countless university students, Calvin was used to being obeyed. But a PhD meant nothing to Alexander the Great.

Minutes later, Avy let the dog back into the house. He galloped past her, paws scrabbling on the hardwood floor, then pivoted back, panting and wagging his wiry body at her feet. Avy bent to scratch his head, then invited him to burrow under the quilt beside her on the couch, the quilt that bore the scent of her mother, and both fell immediately to sleep.

In her exhausted dream, she relived the day when, as a gawky child of eight, she had hiked happily in the footsteps of her mother, Leigh, across a sun-splashed meadow of wildflowers. Her mother called out the names of the native flowers on their way and together they pulled out fistfuls of the invasive species they found—crown vetch, bull thistle, everlasting pea. Triumphantly, Avy threw the weeds to the ground and stomped on them before shoving them into the canvas sack her mother carried.

They finally rested midday in a shady copse of trees. Against the trunk of a paper birch, they looked like bookends holding between them a single black and white volume. While her mother made field notes in a journal, Avy resolved to peel off a sheet of bark big enough to write her own notes on, like Laura Ingalls in *Little House on the Prairie*. A large chunk of bark broke off in her hands, but the fragile inner layer tore when she started to pull it away.

Leigh glanced up from the cup of steaming coffee she had brought in a battered thermos. She closed her field notebook on the bluestem bookmark and leaned toward Avy, who had plopped on the ground beside her. She traced her finger over the faint intermittent lines, flitting like Morse code across the inner layer of the bark in her daughter's hand. "These marks are called lenticels. They allow air to pass through the bark to the inner layers of the tree."

Avy cocked her head, puzzled. "I didn't know trees could breathe." She sprang up, threw her arms around the tree, and pressed her ear against it as if to sense the intake of air into its core. Leigh hid her grin behind another sip of coffee.

Avy flopped back down beside her mother and picked up the chunk of bark she had dropped on the ground. The sturdy outer bark shone white, but beneath it each layer tore away in broken strips to reveal a deeper rosy-brown than the one before. As soft and fragile as the phyllo dough her mother used to make strawberry tarts, the third layer of the inner bark matched the color and smooth texture of Avy's flawless skin.

"If too many layers are pulled from the tree," her mother told her, "that area will become black and hard, a scar that forms over the injury. It's like the scar here on my collarbone. That skin will always be tough, but it protects the tissue beneath from further injury. Pulling off a small piece of the bark like this won't kill the tree, but that spot is damaged and will develop a scar."

Avy looked overhead. There were black patches on the trees all around them. She rose and faced the tree. She gently touched the raw wound where she had pulled the clump of bark away from the trunk. Her eyes closed and her lips moved silently as she bent her head to rest against it. The birch limbs reached down as if to touch her head in a blessing. Avy stood back and looked down on her mother.

"How did you get your scar, Mom?"

"It was an accident." The tenderness in her mother's eyes dimmed, and a hand sprang to the scar on her collarbone. "It happened a long time ago, and it makes me very sad to remember it." Her eyelids closed, like window shades cutting off the brightness of the day. Avy feared that her inquisitiveness had ruined their day, but when her mother lifted her lids sunlight danced in her mother's eyes. Leigh's gentle palms cupped Avy's hands holding the birch bark. "There are tender layers under the surface of my scar, Aviana, just like the layers in this birch bark." Leigh's fingers stroked the soft inner layer of the bark that matched Avy's skin tone. "When I notice my scar now, I try to remember that it covers over the injury that caused it, and protects the soft layers beneath."

Chapter 5

The ragtime tune of Scott Joplin's "The Entertainer" invaded her ears three times before Avy emerged from her Edenic dreamworld and reacted to the cell phone's interruption. She flipped it open while simultaneously wrangling her glasses over her ears. Her watch said 3:13 a.m. Just over an hour ago she had fallen exhausted onto the couch. Now an ebullient voice burst in her ear.

"Avy! Wow! You picked up! It's Andrew. Andrew Chase. From high school."

Andrew. His voice was just as familiar as when he had sat beside her on this very couch.

She hoisted her body up on one elbow, untangled herself from the quilt, and sat up. Alex gave her the stink eye before shifting his aged body into the corner where her legs had recently warmed his back. He gave a final disgruntled snort and closed his filmy eyes. She shifted the cell phone to her right ear.

"Andrew? What on earth?" A cold twilight had replaced her dream's brightness and warmth, and Andrew's anomalous voice in the semidarkness mystified her.

"I'm really sorry to wake you, Avy. It must be after 1:00 a.m. in Denver. I left a message at your dad's house a few hours ago hoping your brother was still in town, but he didn't call back. I didn't know what else to do, so I looked up your phone number out in Colorado and gave it a try. I'm glad I reached you." Avy twisted her body to squint at the message light blinking on the phone in her father's kitchen, causing her back to spasm in pain.

"Andrew. I'm sorry. I didn't catch everything you said." She pressed a fingernail deep into the bridge of her nose, an acupressure trick she used to refocus her thoughts. It wasn't working. "But Jared's moved to Chicago for college. He's prelaw at the University of Chicago." Jared, her little brother who had grown to manhood apart from her. A miasma of regret overcame her for allowing their distance to grow into neglect of their former closeness. She hadn't spoken to him in months. "I have his cell number if you need him. There's no one at home except Dad and Alex."

"Well, that makes it more complicated." She heard a deep breath on the line—counted in-two-three-four, out-two-three-four. Then Andrew's voice again. "Avy, I had to arrest your father tonight." Avy's finger leapt from where it was pressed between her eyes, leaving a thin line of blood across one eyebrow.

"What? But he should be up in his bedroom, sleeping!" She gasped air into her lungs to kick-start her brain cells and twisted to the side to look up the staircase. Moonlight seeped from the open door of her father's bedroom at the top.

"Avy?" Bewilderment overshadowed the usual warmth in his voice. "Are you okay?"

"Oh, crown vetch!" she exploded into the phone. "No, I am not okay!"

There was a long silence on the phone, then—"Where *are* you, Avy?" he asked.

"I've got a mobile phone now, Andrew, tied to my old house number. That's how you reached me. But I'm at Dad's house right now. I got here only an hour ago after driving straight through from Denver. But you're telling me you arrested my dad? What on earth for?"

"So you're in town." He avoided answering her question. "Are you alert enough to drive to the station?"

"Well, I'm certainly not going to fall back to sleep now. I'll be there in ten minutes—unless the station's moved."

"Nope, still on Garfield. I'll be watching for you."

In the police station, the phone went dead. Andrew jerked open the sticky drawer in the old Steelcase desk and fumbled around for his Tic Tacs.

⸻ ◆ ⸻

Avy flipped the phone closed and dropped it into the open backpack on the floor. She wondered what else could happen in twenty-four hours. She rose, hoisted the pack, and tucked the quilt around the dog, so at least *he* could sleep.

She stepped back out into the cold night, started the car, and headed downtown. She was awake enough now to replay her endless day in disjointed snatches. All she remembered of the last hour's drive was the bossy GPS voice, advising her to return to the highlighted route before she punched the off button. And all she wanted to do was crawl back under the quilt where she could collapse, like a lost starling in an abandoned nest cavity.

⸻ ◆ ⸻

She spotted Andrew standing by the window of the police station, peering out. Looking for her. Her head fell back against the headrest. It had been years since they'd spoken, even longer since they'd seen each other. She'd left without saying goodbye. How could she face him now, after all this time and in these circumstances? She swiveled the rearview and swiped a finger under each eye. She squinted though the windshield and the light falling snow. He was still scanning the darkness outside. No sense in putting this off. She swung open the door and stepped onto the cold asphalt. Andrew sprinted to open the station door as she marched in. A freezing wind accompanied her.

Without preamble, she demanded, "Now tell me what on earth is going on!"

"Okay," he said, indicating a pair of leatherette chairs against a wall. "Let's sit down and I'll tell you everything."

"I might fall asleep if I sit down, so just start talking." Avy paced the floor of the small office, thumbs and middle fingers framing her taut face from brow to jawline. She glanced once at a solid door at the back of the station where she assumed her father was snoring away, then dragged her attention back to Andrew.

"Okay," he repeated. He rounded the corner of his desk to barricade himself against her snappishness and dropped into his ancient metal desk chair. "A call came in around 9:45 from a security guard at the mall. Two young girls reported they were walking through the parking lot from the theater. Security said they were looking for a brother that was supposed to pick them up. When a black Buick rolled up near them, they said the guy put down the window and called them over. One of the girls held back, but the other went up to the passenger window to see what he wanted."

Avy stopped pacing and leaned her weight against Andrew's desk. Her father had purchased a black Buick the year she left. She absently noted the box from Marge's Donut Den in the trash can, the overlapping circles of coffee stains on the desk blotter, and a photo of Andrew and his dad in hiking gear on the edge of a cliff—shortly before his father's fatal heart attack. She lost the track of his story.

"Sorry, Andrew. I'm having a hard time focusing. Start over with the girl walking up to the car."

"Well, when she got up to the window and leaned down to see what he wanted, the first thing she noticed was a large doll on the passenger seat." He stopped, wiped a hand across his brow, then took a deep breath and resumed. "Then she saw that the driver's pants were unzipped and his hands were—"

Avy reared up, holding both palms in front of him. Her dark eyes flashed. "No! Hold it right there. This is crazy! He may be many things, but my father is not a pervert!" Her eyes sparked a warning.

Andrew's department-issue chair squeaked harshly in the charged silence as he leaned forward against the force of her anger, his hands gripping the armrests, and pushed himself up. He'd have to show her. He strode three steps to a locker and spun the combination.

"You never could get the combination right in biology lab." She recalled the familiar sight from ten years back. Andrew's shoulders had broadened since then, she noticed, the blue shirt taut across his shoulder blades. And he moved with unfamiliar authority. She circled the corner of his desk, crossing the invisible barrier he had set up. By the time she twirled his empty chair around and sank into it, he had the locker open. He turned resolutely, clutching an evidence box, and deposited it on the desk before her.

"This is what we took from his car. And from his person."

He lifted the lid. Avy leaned forward, accompanied by the squeal of the chair, to peer into the cardboard box. On top of the contents, a large cloth doll spilled out of a plastic evidence bag.

"That's Melinda! My mom gave her to me. I thought Dad threw her out years ago with all of Mom's other stuff."

Avy jumped to her feet and slid the doll from the bag before Andrew could protest. She hugged the shabby thing to her chest for only the length of a heartbeat. Then she grimaced, held the doll at arm's length, and reared back. The soft contours of her doll were now misshapen in her hands and a gamy smell, like body odor or worse, penetrated her nostrils. The doll's once colorfully striped jumper was torn and dingy. Avy's face had turned into a mask of grief.

"She was my best friend. I carried her everywhere, and then, after Mom died, she disappeared." She gazed plaintively at the doll. "And her blouse was white, not this vomit-colored rag." Avy's mouth pursed and she let the doll drop onto Andrew's desk blotter.

Andrew nodded brusquely, avoiding her wounded eyes. From the evidence box, he withdrew an empty Tanqueray bottle, a mahogany-colored leather wallet shaped to the curve of a back pocket, a set of keys on a ring flaunting the Grand River State University logo, and a battered briefcase stuffed with dog-eared magazines.

"His alcohol level was point one six, twice the legal limit, and the open bottle still contained a few drops. He's sleeping it off in the back. I've been keeping an eye on him with the camera." He pointed Avy's attention to the small image in the monitor suspended from the ceiling, which sloughed paint flecks like dandruff onto the floor. Lying on a narrow cot, a man covered in a charcoal-colored blanket faced the gray cinder-block wall. She propelled herself around the desk to stop beneath the video monitor, looking up at the inclined screen.

"That looks like his back alright." Her voice grated between clenched teeth. "I had the opportunity to see it often enough." Her eyes remained fixed on the still image.

"I knew he liked to drink," Avy mused, her clutched fists pressed into her sides. "I always thought it was a bit of an affectation, you know? The brilliant professor sipping his brandy at the end of a grueling day of dispensing wisdom. But I never knew him to get drunk." Befuddlement clouded her eyes as she pivoted from the monitor to face Andrew.

"The other girl memorized the license plate number and the make and color of the car before they ran off and found the security guy. Your dad was still right where they told us they saw him, passed out, when I drove up. He continued, eyes averted, "I had no idea who I was coming to pick up until I got him out of the car. I recognized him in spite of how he's changed in ten years. I'm sorry, Avy, but I had to bring him in for a DUI"—he paused—"and indecent exposure—although I was relieved to see that his pants were zipped when I held him up against the car."

"Tree of Heaven!" Avy dropped back into Andrew's chair and shut her eyes. Her head rocked slowly on the back of the chair, her hands pressed against her forehead.

Andrew eased onto the edge of his desk in front of her, knocking over the photo, and drew a breath. Avy shifted, the top half of her body curling over her lap. Her elbows dropped to her knees and her hands slid down to cover her face.

"His alcohol level has dropped now to below the legal limit, so I can release him into your custody if you're able to get him to court by three this afternoon for arraignment." She gave no response. Andrew continued. "Do you know if he has a lawyer? Otherwise I'll call the public defender's office as soon as they're open in the morning."

"I'll see if I can locate the lawyer he had years ago when I was still at home." Her palms muffled the response. "I'll let you know."

"Listen, Avy. It's still dark out. The girls have no idea who he is. And I don't think they want to press charges. In fact, I got the feeling they thought it was kinda funny." He shrugged his shoulders when Avy swiveled her head and rolled her eyes in his direction. "Look. No one else needs to know about this for now. He'll just have to pay a fine, I think, for the DUI. It's a first offense. And if the girls don't press charges, the indecent exposure goes away. Since no one else witnessed what happened, it would be their word against his anyway, but you should still have a lawyer."

"I've been away a long time," she murmured. She rolled her head back and forth in her palms, then lifted her chin to release her strained neck muscles. Andrew waited for her to continue. The silence stretched.

"So," he ventured at last, "what are you doing back in town? It's good to see you after so long, despite all this." He dared to touch her shoulder.

The vertebrae, scalloped beside her dark braid, snapped into place to raise her head and shake off Andrew's palm.

She rose to face him, leaning in. "I'm *not* back!" Defiance burned in her eyes. "It took everything I had to *leave* his house. I've made myself into the strong, independent woman I am, and I won't be dragged back into his life! I'm on my way to New York. Long story. I just stopped here in Berndtbridge to get some sleep— big mistake."

"I'm sorry." Andrew backed away, palming his hands in defense. "Well, he needs to show up in court by three. I can keep him here if you don't want to take him back to the house."

"No." Avy released a sigh. "Sorry, Andrew. I didn't mean to jump on you. If we can get him into my car, I'll take him home."

"Sure you want to do that? It's no problem—him staying here. You can just take off for New York and he won't even know you were here. Remember what he's been accused of, even if he's not charged."

"I'm a big girl, Andrew. I can handle it," she retorted, staring at the monitor, at the man lying as still as a boulder. "Better to get him out of here while it's still dark than in the light of day."

Chapter 6

Was she dreaming? No. The footsteps continued their slow approach, thump-grunt, thump-grunt, thump-grunt. "Whoa!" A man's muffled voice. She struggled to wake and face the intruder. At her feet, Alex snorted at the sound of creaking floorboards—the landing at the turn of the stairs, she realized. She dragged open her eyes to see a fold of fabric in front of her face, partially obstructing her vision. She was lying on the sofa, she recalled, cocooned in her mother's quilt. The dog shifted at the sound, rolling his bony torso across her ankles, and propped his head on the arm of the sofa at her feet. The eyes of both of them were trained on the man on the stairs—her father, clinging to the newel post for balance before navigating the last three stairs. She wasn't ready to face him. Her eyes closed to slits beneath her eyelashes, and she pretended to sleep.

Calvin Lehrer straightened and rubbed at his rheumy eyes, staring at the mound on the sofa. She breathed deeply, emitting a believable snore, as she watched him approach. He shuffled closer, bent down over her, and grunted, "Gaelle!" He tottered backward, reeling against the arm of an overstuffed chair, and toppled into it. "It's been a long time," he mumbled. "Wonder what the hell brought her back here after all these years."

Avy moaned and shifted, as if in sleep. She twisted away from him and the hurt of the name he used—Gaelle. Even after all these years, she thought, he wouldn't use her rightful name. She curled her body deep into the back of the couch. Alex took the opportunity to press himself deeper into the curve of her body.

"My head," her father whined. "Feels like someone mistook it for a bass drum." She heard his struggle—grunting and mumbling—to get up from the chair. "What I need is a little 'hair of the dog.'" He shuffled into the kitchen.

The door beneath the sink opened and banged against the adjacent cupboard. She could hear mumbling and scrabbling among the contents of the recess, and then a clang as a tower of empty cans toppled onto the linoleum floor.

"Damn it!" her father growled. "I guess coffee will have to do instead, since my Tanqueray seems to have disappeared." She heard the sound of a metal can being dragged from a cabinet and set on the counter, the plastic lid being pried off, tap water running into the glass pot, then sloshing into the reservoir of the Mr. Coffee.

But the dog's snoring soon lulled her back to sleep.

A greasy odor, mingled with bursts of dog breath, roused her. She traced the first scent to the kitchen—where her father stood at the stove, humming tunelessly while scraping the metal spatula across a frying pan—and the second to the tongue lapping the drool from her open mouth.

"Get back, you stupid mutt!" she rasped, shoving the eager terrier away. She nearly fell off the couch, her legs tangled in the quilt.

Undeterred, Alex leapt back onto her chest, barking an exuberant greeting in her face. Resigned to his irrepressible energy, even at his advanced age, she flipped him onto his back for a belly rub. "Well, at least *you're* happy to see me, old buddy," she whispered. "Sorry I called you stupid. What do you think about the old man? Got any suggestions for how I should handle him?" In response, Alex bounded from her chest to the floor and skidded across the kitchen linoleum to her father's feet, without missing a beat in his incessant barking. Avy rose up slowly on one elbow, disentangled herself from the quilt, and sank back into the cratered cushion. She rotated her neck and shoulders to ease the cramped muscles. A familiar sharp pain attacked her back as she scooted to the edge of the sofa.

Only a few hours ago, she had stumbled with her father over the threshold into the darkened house, arms around each other's shoulders like old drinking buddies staggering down the sidewalk. Avy had lugged him up the stairs as he doggedly sang "Roll Out the Barrel," while Alex inserted himself between their feet. She'd backed her father up against his unmade bed and guided the heavy descent of his rear end onto the squeaking springs. There, she held him upright by his collar long enough to wrestle his rank-smelling shirt over his head. He toppled backward; the sleeves furled to his wrists and caught at the buttoned cuffs. She held the shirttail taut in a one-sided tug-of-war and stared numbly down at her father's slack face lolling back on the bed.

She gave up, released the shirt, and his hands landed like a rock in his crotch. A loud grunt was his only response.

Alex had beaten her down the stairs but allowed her space enough to crawl back under the quilt, where she passed out on the musty couch.

Now dust motes sifted down through the prism of sunlight that trickled through the single windowpane high in the front door. The sight recalled the previous night's newly fallen snow. She gathered her legs under her and stood, dropping the quilt in a tangle on the floor next to the worn backpack. She resigned herself to confronting her father; no sense putting it off. She followed Alex's path into the kitchen, leaned against the doorframe, and considered the man.

Did he even remember what happened last night? She looked at his back, and at the messy kitchen, and wondered how he had gotten into the state he was in. It looked like he had given up on life.

Everything in the once-bright kitchen, where she had felt such warmth working beside her mother, was painted with grime and neglect. The tulip-patterned wallpaper had dulled under the layers of grease and smoke, so that it felt as though the flowers bent beneath a perpetual rain cloud. Encrusted dishes filled the sink. A broken flowerpot, holding a desiccated stem stretching up forlornly from the dry clods of dirt, sat abandoned on the windowsill. The calendar on the wall remained open to last May. A brown banana attracting a cloud of fruit flies, used tissues, and a once-clear drinking glass now serving as a petri dish for a Salmonella colony, shared the surface of the kitchen table with a bag of Epsom salts, a bottle of Tums, and a toenail clipper—recently used, as evidenced by a pile of clippings atop unread mail, on a chair. News clippings and food wrappers spilled onto the floor.

She sagged against the doorframe to see how the place, and the man, were falling apart. He looked much older than his sixty-three years. He was drinking too much, neglecting things, and she still couldn't fathom what had happened last night.

Her father hummed a meaningless tune at the stove, his back to her. A new bald spot glowed like a dim light shining behind a scrim of thinning hair. Limp ebony waves, sprinkled with silver, brushed his bathrobe collar. The solid reality of her prematurely aging father stood in sharp contrast to the bright memories of her mother that had been reawakened by the dream.

She coveted those long-lost days before her mother became ill. When she was alive, Avy felt connected to someone who loved and delighted in her. She had not needed or missed her father's attention, the attention he had showered, presumably, on his wife, Leigh—otherwise, how could she have married him? And he had fussed over Avy's sister, the beautiful Auralei, who looked so much like their mother. But most devotedly, he doted on his beloved son, Jared. In *her* life, though, he loomed like an imposing boulder, a part of her landscape, but not a part of the animate world she and her mother shared.

When her mother died three years after Jared was born, twelve-year-old Avy found that mourning her mother was like stoking a seductive fire. She was warmed and comforted by the memories as she drew near. But, like drawing too close to a fire, the intensity of those memories could consume her with pain.

On her closet floor she'd amassed a small cache of her mother's possessions. Her mother's hiking boots cradled the woolen socks in a kindling nest that kept the fire alive. And her nature sketches added fuel for the memories' flame.

She remembered predawn excursions to Point Pelee National Park in search of the red-necked grebe migrating through Lake Erie all the way from Alaska; tracking coyotes through the borders and the alleys of Detroit; spying, through her mother's binoculars, on the endangered Kirtland's warbler feeding nestlings in a remote jack pine forest in northern Michigan.

The binoculars had hung from her closet door, yet one day they disappeared, along with the boots and most of her mother's other personal possessions. Avy stowed away her growing realization that love and grief, joy and pain, wove and pressed themselves together like her mother's nubby woolen socks.

She'd managed to hide the socks inside her pillowcase, where the woolly smell and rough texture fueled her memories at night. She claimed laundry duty—not that anyone else would fight her for it—to avoid having them found by her father.

And years later, when she packed surreptitiously to escape, she tucked the socks and some clothes into her mother's old backpack, along with the cash she had managed to squirrel away. The same sturdy one that now sat on the floor by the sofa.

After the death of her mother, she had tried to reach out to her father, but found only a distant man—a man who seemed never to know what to think of her, what to do with her. She became invisible.

———————

Invisible. As she was now, staring once again at her father's back.

"Gaelle," he said finally, fussing over a frying pan on the stove, not bothering even to look at her. "What brings you here?" Gaelle—the old name he had reverted to calling her, which she hadn't heard in ten years. She understood that her parents had disagreed, but that her mother stood firm, refusing to back down on the name she had her heart set on—Aviana, "the way of grace," she'd been told, "to signify hope, and lightness—like a bird!" Her mother always called her Aviana. But her father, if he called her anything at all, used only Gaelle. When she studied German in high school, she had learned its meaning—"stranger"—and felt again the sting of his rejection.

"I decided on the spur of the moment to stop by," she said, stepping into the kitchen and the current reality. The image of the ghostly owl careened back into her mind and she banished it just as quickly. "I've left Denver. I'm on my way to New York." Still, her father busied himself at the stove. She went on. "I have a promising job prospect with a major hospital in Albany. It's a great opportunity. I would start in two weeks."

"Oh," her father said. "You were in Denver, too? I didn't know."

That was a lie, she knew. She had called him seven years ago to let him know where she was and how to reach her. But he never did.

Automatically, she began the Lamaze breathing she had learned in her obstetrics rotation in nursing school. The technique always worked in ticklish situations at the hospital—although it had failed her that day two weeks ago. Avy wished she had known it as an adolescent.

She barely held her disappointment in check. He hadn't really changed in relation to her—she was still Gaelle to him.

"Look, Dad, you can't make me feel guilty now for not coming home in all these years." Sleep deprivation prevented her from controlling her words. Rekindled after ten years, smoldering resentment flared, escaping her meticulously maintained firebreak, the distance she had kept between her scalded heart and the arsonist before her now.

"You never cared if I existed before I left, except as someone to take care of the house and Jared. Why would I come back to where I wasn't wanted? You're the one who always told others, 'Go where you're appreciated, not just tolerated.' You barely tolerated me, so I found a place where I mattered, and I did very well for myself!" She quickly smothered the flicker of recognition that she had not, after all, been appreciated enough for the longed-for promotion. She resolved right then that she would be well respected in her new home.

Her face burned with the fire of her long-simmering bitterness toward her father. Tears stung her eyes, but she refused to let them fall on the flame of her anger.

"You fawned over Auralei like she was a princess—until your precious little son was born! No wonder she took off when you turned all your attention to Jared."

Jared. The memory of her sweet little brother threatened to disarm her. Little Jared, with his ebony curls and chestnut eyes that mirrored their father's, found the crevices into the man's heart. And only through Jared, she thought, could she hope to be seen, to be valued, to belong with someone again.

In those early months of her grief, it had fallen to her, since their schools were in adjacent buildings, to shepherd Jared to and from preschool. She recalled the spicy-sweet scent of her little brother's dark curls those first few days of fall, when he'd clung fiercely to her neck in the preschool entry. She refused to care about the detention she received in her first week of seventh grade when Jared's tears made her late to school three days in a row. Her only aim was to comfort and nurture the little boy that their mother no longer could. Jared required all of her attention, and she tried to care for him as she knew his mother would have done. She read him to sleep with the stories of *Frog and Toad* and *Goodnight Moon*. She taught him all she had learned from their mother about trees and animals, flowers, birds, and rocks. She kissed away his fears.

That precious intimacy, the love of and from her brother that gave her life new meaning, ended abruptly in the spring of her junior year.

Their father had decided it was time for eight-year-old Jared to learn to play baseball like other boys his age, and to stop being coddled by his sister. So he signed the boy up for Little League, in spite of Jared's fears.

Because her father's classes that semester kept him busy in the late afternoons, it was her job, now that she could drive, to pick him up afterward from the ballpark. She had intended to get to her brother's games in time to give him the support the other boys had from their parents, but on his first day, her reshelving job at the library kept her until 4:30.

She raced from the library and pulled into the parking lot in time to see Jared slouching from the field. Loping from the car, she reached the bleachers just as the coach rounded the fence at a run and whipped Jared around by the shoulder. He got up in the boy's face spitting out anger in front of the watchers in the bleachers.

Avy shouted over the coach's rant, catching Jared by surprise. The boy whirled and threw himself at her, knocking her to the ground. His twisted face, burning with humiliation, hung over her. He shrieked, "Shut up! You're not my mother!"

The coach yanked Jared up by his shirt and shook him. "The kid's gotta toughen up," he shouted at Avy, who lay stunned on the grass. He slapped her little brother's taut buttocks and walked Jared by the nape of the neck back to the field. Taunting laughter reached her as she gathered herself up. Jared's new teammates stood lined up at the fence, watching and jeering. His open palm crashed into the chain link backstop next to the nearest face.

"Break's over," yelled the coach, and the boys scattered back out to the field, while Jared was plunked, seething, on the bench. She imagined the diamond-shaped red welts on that soft palm, and realized she was massaging her own with her thumb.

She could still feel the softness of his palm in hers, but she realized he had stopped holding her hand months before. He was deserting her too, just like the rest of the family. First, her mother, then Auralei. And now Jared. She sat on a cold boulder by the parking lot to wait till the game finished, and she sensed her body fading away, disappearing into the air, no longer of any substance or use.

When her brother was born, she was nine and Auralei twelve, already moving confidently from precious childhood into adolescent beauty. When their father became so obsessed with his newborn son that he ignored even her sister, Auralei simply turned away from her family—including Avy. But teenaged boys were more than willing to affirm Auralei's place of entitlement in the world. She had disappeared into high school, where she was welcomed into a cadre of beautiful friends and practiced "catch and release" with a string of boyfriends. Her father noticed her only when she was suspended for three days and he was forced to pay attention. Avy, on the other hand, managed to avoid his attention by always doing what was expected.

———◆——

Even now, her instinct was to recant the accusations she had just spewed out. She had never before spoken up to him like that.

But her father spoke again from his stakeout at the stove. "I'm having eggs. You can fix your own, now that you've finally stopped snoring," he said, sliding the contents of the frying pan onto a chipped plate.

He had simply ignored her diatribe, she realized. Her harsh words meant nothing to him!

With her anger still burning, the bitterness of her hurt tasted like vinegar on her tongue and backflowed into her throat and nostrils. She needed coffee to wash it away. She felt the glass pot. The coffee was still warm, so she poured the dregs into a relatively clean mug that she found at the back of a cabinet and added hot water from the tap. Then she took a ragged breath and steeled herself to confront him about his behavior at the mall and its consequences.

"Father," she began—

"I don't have any bacon," he said. "It's on the list of a hundred and one foods forbidden by the doctor." He turned from the counter. "But then, you look like you could do without it yourself." After an appraising stare at her solid figure, he turned with his breakfast toward the overloaded table and shuffled past her. The surface of the slimy eggs shone like congealed motor oil on the plate.

"Cabomba! Those eggs are spoiled!" She stepped back, aghast as the sulfurous smell wafted over her. Her father's hands trembled under the slight weight of the plate.

"I can't eat fried eggs, Dad," she managed. "And neither should you if your doctor's cutting fat and cholesterol out of your diet." She slipped the plate from his hands, turned, and slid the slimy eggs into the garbage disposal.

"What the—" The grinding of the disposal cut off his objection. His eyes glared at her as she turned, empty plate still shining with grease. He opened his mouth, then abruptly dropped sideways into a chair at the kitchen table, shoving papers off to join the others on the floor, and stared at his clenched fists. Before her was a defiant man, as he had always been, but now he was bluffing his way through life.

"The eggs are spoiled, Dad! What were you thinking? I can't believe what I'm finding since I got here. This place is a disaster!"

She took over mechanically, resuming her old role of providing sustenance, keeping the family's body and soul together and trying to avoid conflict. She needed to hold her anger in check and manage to get him to court today. It would require a firm hand and self-control. She could do this, she reminded herself. She had remade herself into a strong, competent woman in the last decade. Just because she was back under his roof, she wouldn't let him resume control of her. *She* was in control now. She straightened, looked down at him with his greasy hair and disheveled robe, and said with inarguable self-assurance, "How about I fix some oatmeal instead? You still like it with raisins and brown sugar? Then we need to talk."

Chapter 7

At the kitchen table, she leaned her chin on her hands, folded as if in prayer. Her father had refused to respond to her or acknowledge the previous night's actions, silently eating his oatmeal and chasing it with bitter coffee. Then he headed for the sofa, crawled under the quilt, and turned away from her. He hadn't moved since. The light from the ceiling fixture overhead shone feebly on the debris strewn about her on the table and overflowing onto the chairs and floor beneath. She reached for the nearly empty Tums bottle and popped another between her teeth. The kitchen phone rang, and she lifted the grimy receiver to her ear.

"Hello. Avy Lehrer here."

"Monfort-Cadge Law, Cadge speaking. I understand that you need representation at the courthouse today at 3:00 o'clock. Is that correct?"

"Yes. It's for my father, Calvin Lehrer. Dale Monfort has represented him in the past at the time of my mother's death, and I was hoping he might be available."

"I'm sorry, but Mr. Monfort is out of the country at this time. May I be of assistance instead?"

"Actually, that might be preferable." She took a deep breath. "My father was arrested last night but released into my custody. He's been accused of driving while intoxicated and for indecent exposure. It's hard to imagine he would have exposed himself if he hadn't been drunk, but I've been gone for years and I'm finding him quite changed. The arresting officer, Andrew Chase, said Dad would maybe only have to pay a fine—that he wasn't actually driving at the time, just sitting in the car. But I'm worried that it could mean jail time if the parents of the girls who saw him decide to pursue it. I arrived in town late last night, only to be confronted with this nightmare. I don't know what to do. Can you take his case?"

"I'll meet you and your father there. Be prepared to pay a fine as high as a thousand dollars if the DUI was a first offense, but I'll keep him from any more jail time. If the girl or her family *do* decide to press charges, since he was drunk, we can argue he didn't realize what he was doing and didn't intend to expose himself."

"I'm beginning to wonder if he may have intended just that. Like I said, he's not the man he was ten years ago. I don't really know him anymore." She added, "But the officer said it would be a matter of 'he said-she said,' since there were no other witnesses."

"Well, keep all that to yourself and let me do my work. I'll see you there."

"Alright. Thank you."

He hung up, but she held on to the receiver, slowly knocking it against her head as she observed her father's inert form. Finally, she dropped it back in the cradle, crossed "call lawyer" off her list, and went to his study to look for her father's checkbook.

She returned to the kitchen with it, sorted through the mess on the table, and tossed dried bread crusts and junk mail into the garbage along with the scattered cans littering the floor. She set aside unopened bills to be dealt with later. From under the sink, she retrieved a desiccated sponge and a bottle of dish soap that had tipped over, spilling most of its contents. She plugged the sink and filled it with steaming water, loading crusted silverware, glasses and plates in to soak. Then she scrubbed the table and the phone receiver for good measure. She scowled at the phone.

First, she would call Jared in Chicago. Surely, he was aware of their father's decline.

<hr>

"Geez, Dad. I was asleep! What time is it?"

"It's nearly 11:00 a.m. here. And this isn't Dad."

"Avy? What are you doing on Dad's phone? Are you there?"

"That should be obvious since you're hearing me on his phone line and he never bothered to get a mobile. I'm sitting at his kitchen table, in complete chaos," she said. "I was on my way to New York for an interview for a new position, and I made the mistake of stopping here to get some sleep. Dad's got himself in a mess."

"Hah! Going anywhere near Dad is definitely a mistake. I was glad to get out of there. By the way, it's nice to hear your voice again after so many months."

"Yeah, you too. I considered detouring to see you in Chicago, but I was anxious to get to Albany. I thought I could do it in one stretch—big mistake. I must have zoned out and I found myself in Michigan. I nearly drove off an embankment to my death. But never mind that."

"Okaaay. So, what's going on with Dad?"

"Oh—nothing much. He just got busted last night. Only driving under the influence and indecent exposure."

"Dad? No way!"

"Oh yes, way. My old friend Andrew's the one who arrested him, and I dragged the old man home from the station early this morning on the promise I would get him to the courthouse this afternoon and pay the fine. Could be up to a thousand bucks. Not to mention the lawyer's fee to keep him out of jail."

"Oh, you really stepped in the shit with both feet, didn't you?" She heard stifled laughter.

"Yeah. Very funny, Jared. Listen, that's just the immediate problem. There's more. The house is a disaster and this morning he cooked up some rotten eggs, expecting to eat them. He's losing it! Didn't you notice anything wrong before you left for Chicago? Have you been back to check on him?"

"Hey, take it down a notch! Where have *you* been the last ten years? Off doing your own thing; no worries about the old man or the little brother you left behind to fend for himself. How do you think it was for *me* growing up?"

"But you had him all to yourself, and he adored you!"

"What are you talking about? He didn't *adore* me. He smoth-ered me—trying to mold and shape me into his likeness. Listen. Have you heard of the latest Mike Myers movie—*Austin Powers: The Spy Who Shagged Me?*"

She didn't bother to answer. She hated crudeness. And she hadn't been out to a movie . . . well, in years.

"No? A bunch of guys from the house went to see it the first weekend we were here. It's best seen after playing beer pong—it's that stupid. I bring it up because there's a character in it, a clone of Dr. Evil that he calls Mini-Me. That's exactly what Dad wanted from me—a mini version of himself."

Her head swirled with the unfamiliar titles—beer pong? Dr. Evil? Mini-Me? She realized she was way out of touch.

"He wanted me to follow in his footsteps. Education was everything to him, you know. Why do you think I did so well in school? He would have killed me if I hadn't been in the top five. The fact that I was accepted at the University of Chicago proved I was worthy to be his son, that his intelligence genes had been passed along. I don't know how you escaped his badgering, but I'm working very hard to rid myself of the image and expectation he had for me. You and Auralei were lucky to escape when you did. Like I said, I was glad to finally get the hell out of there."

"I had no idea, Jared. I envied you. I felt so lost after Mom died, and Dad paid no attention to me."

"Yeah. Well, I don't even remember Mom. You did a pretty decent job of mothering me, though. I owe you for that."

Avy gulped. Her hand was moist where she gripped the phone receiver. She sat back in the chair and felt the muscles tighten in her throat.

"You were all I had left," she murmured.

There were only the sounds of the clock ticking and quiet breathing on the other end of the phone.

"Listen," he said, "I'm planning to come home over Christmas break, but I won't be making a habit of a pilgrimage back to the old homestead. Yeah, I knew he was letting things go, but I didn't think much of it. I'm not much of a neat freak myself. It was just us two guys—well three if you count Alex—for so many years. I guess we just turned into slobs. Hey—is Alex okay?"

"Yes, your precious dog is as feisty as ever. But I'm really worried about Dad. We need to do something."

"You're overreacting, Avy. You said he was drunk last night, so he probably didn't know what he was doing. And he just didn't notice the eggs were bad this morning. How *would* he know anyway? How can you tell if eggs are rotten? He'll be fine. I'll check up on him next month, but he'll be okay."

"I don't think so, Jared."

"Well, what do you expect me to do? I don't plan to give up my life—now that I finally have one—to babysit him."

"I'm not *expecting* anything, Jared. I just need to talk this out with you and Auralei."

"Ah, so you haven't talked to our big sister yet, eh? Good luck with that. But I think you just happened to catch Dad at a particularly bad time. He never drank much when I was home—at least not that I saw. He just needs to lose the hangover and take care of whatever it was that happened last night. He'll be fine. Trust me. Now tell me about this new job opportunity of yours."

"Never mind that right now. We'll talk again soon." She wouldn't get any support from her brother. He had run away just as she had years ago.

"Okay, sis. It was good to hear your voice."

"Back atcha, bro. It's been too long. I'm happy that you seem to have started on your own path. Good luck with that."

Fresh from a hurried shower, she peeked over the banister to see that her father still slept on the sofa. Then she dressed in her interview suit, retrieved from the car. Her makeup was in the bottom of the canvas backpack, still lying on the living room floor by the sofa. She didn't want to risk waking her father before she had to, so she left her face bare and braided her wet hair, settling it on a folded towel down her back to keep it from dampening her blouse.

Taking a deep breath, she opened the door to her father's bedroom. The bedspread still held the impression of his body where she had dumped him in the middle of the night. His soiled clothes lay on the floor by the chair in the corner. Somehow, he'd managed to untangle himself from the shirt and pants and put on his tattered robe before coming downstairs that morning. She strode to the window and pulled on the shade to release it. Dust billowed, but the shade didn't snap up. She tried the other window and found this shade partially torn from the roller.

"How can he live like this?"

She stepped to the closet and pulled the light cord. The bulb glowed on her father's drab clothing. She pulled out a suit, shirt, and tie, and laid it out on the bed. Shoes, socks—she refused to look for underwear. He'd have to do that himself.

They had to be at the courthouse in less than two hours. Somehow, she had to get him to understand that what he had done last night had landed him in trouble. Big trouble.

She wanted to tell him 'actions have consequences.' That's what he had drilled into them as kids back when the shoe was on the other foot. She was beginning to think it would have been so much better to have left him in Andrew's custody and kept driving east. Why did she have to be so obstinate and take responsibility for him?

She released a gust of air through pursed lips, straightened her shoulders, and closed the bedroom door behind her. Somehow, she would see this through. Then she'd be back on the road.

Chapter 8

He hadn't spoken to her since pleading guilty to the DUI and paying the fine at the courthouse. The judge waived the indecent exposure, since the girl's family declined to press charges and no one had shown up at the courthouse to corroborate the incident. Her father hadn't looked in her direction or acknowledged her presence after leaving the courtroom and getting into her car. They had stopped at the police station to retrieve his belongings from the officer on the day shift. Her father didn't respond to her as she passed him his keys.

Avy couldn't bring herself to exit the car. Her hands still gripped the steering wheel as she watched him fumble with the front door. She had locked it behind them when they headed to the courthouse. He rummaged in his pocket for the key and jammed it in the lock.

When the door slammed behind him, Avy lowered her head between her hands on the wheel; her body shook with frustration. Only when the spasms stopped and she could release the steering wheel did she take a deep breath, open the door with a defiant shove, and step out onto the driveway.

Pausing at the closed front door, she could hear music—the piano pounding out "Won't You Come Home, Bill Bailey." Hughie Cannon was her father's favorite among the ragtime pioneers. She eased open the door. Her father's legs practically danced beneath the piano bench as his fingers flew over the keys. She stood rooted to the oak floor.

The piano needed tuning, but in a way, the off-key playing seemed to match the ragtime melody, and the incongruity of the cheerful music with the bitter rancor of the afternoon began to unlock her taut facial muscles. Her fingers twitched with the memory of lessons her father had begun to drill into her at the age of nine. "The Cat Came Back" began to play in her head and, as if he read her mind, her father launched into the song that had tormented her as a girl. He'd made her play it over and over while he growled out the lyrics. It was meant to be a humorous children's song, but she'd been repulsed by the words. Everyone was trying to kill a poor cat, but each of *them*, instead, died in turn!

She wondered why he was playing these songs about coming back, coming home, and dying. Was he trying to tell her he wished her dead? Or that she'd been dead to him? Or just that she was stupid for coming back?

She'd never reached the proficiency on the piano that her father wished for her, and she had grown weary of his criticism of this, too. On her own, she had mastered James Taylor's "Fire and Rain." Learning the sweet, sad song was a wordless tribute to her mother, who had loved Taylor's mellow voice and played his music over and over. When Avy had begun to play it proudly on the piano for her father one day, he crashed his palms down on the keys to stop her. She responded by slamming the fallboard over the keys, not caring if she smashed his fingers, and refused to make music ever again. No amount of punishment could make her sit back down on that bench. But no punishment had come. The old upright had remained shut and still.

Yet here was her father, suddenly rocking out the music as if he had never stopped playing. Maybe he hadn't. She had been wrong to think that the music showed he was in a better mood. No, he had chosen that particular children's song to punish her—for today, for coming back, for anything and everything. She crossed the room and climbed the stairs to the accompaniment of a jarring rendition of "Chopsticks."

She rested her hand on the cold chrome doorknob of her old room, where she had passed so many lonely hours—despite sharing it with Auralei. But she was spent—both mind and body squeezed of thought, feeling, and will. She needed to sleep; Her old bed, at least, would welcome her. After that she would try again to call her sister.

She kicked off her shoes, threw back the spread, and tumbled onto the bed. Dust motes swirled through the one narrow beam of sunlight peeking past the edge of the blinds. When she dragged the spread over herself, the odor of neglect assailed her, but she burrowed her face into the pillow anyway, willing her mind into oblivion.

In Avy's dream, her mother glided several steps ahead of her through the wildflower meadow. The sun shimmered off her bare arms as they swung gracefully, brushing aside the grasses that reached into the air above her head. Avy followed in her path, laughing and singing. She had never seen such an abundance in the meadow, heard such joy bubbling from the nearby stream. She wiped perspiration from her forehead. The sun was so bright! She spun, arms out-flung in an exuberant dance. But when she stopped spinning, the wildflowers and grasses had sprung back across the path and her mother was no longer in sight. And now she spied chicory springing up around her, and goatsbeard. Everlasting pea and bittersweet nightshade circled her ankles.

"Motherwort!" she screamed.

"Keep up, Aviana!" her mother called from a distance. "I don't have much time. Clumps of bark are dropping and the birch tree is dying!"

A wind had risen and pushed the clouds across the sun, bending the bull thistle to catch in her hair.

"I'm trying, Mom! Wait for me!" No answer.

"Banish! Be gone!" Avy cried at the encroaching plants. Tears ran down her face as she ripped the thistles from her hair. Frantically, she tore at the vines climbing up her legs. Her hands came away red with blood and the juice of the poisonous nightshade berries, but she was free. She ran, unable to orient herself by the sun, still hidden behind scudding clouds. Rain began to pelt her skin and she realized she was naked. Still, she ran.

Finally she spied a towering birch and broke through into a mossy bog, her feet squooshing in mud and rock snot. Her mother stood, bucking the wind at the foot of the birch, arms raised to its whipping branches, intoning sounds Avy could not understand. White bark fell in clumps around her, building up like sand at the bottom of an hourglass.

"Mother!" she called. Her mother turned, her face white as the tree, and her eyes as black and empty as the scars that marred its bark. Then she sank, as if melting, down into the bark-pile, and was obscured from Avy's view.

A sudden stillness descended over her, her feet still mired in the bog. She struggled to uproot them and staggered to the base of the naked tree. Hands scrabbling in the dry bark, she searched, but her mother had disappeared. Brittle brown heart-shaped leaves drifted down around her, catching in her hair. She collapsed, weeping at the foot of the tree.

As her tears abated, she noticed that her back felt warm and a soft intermittent breeze like a breath on her neck seemed to penetrate to her bones. The sensation was as if she were held close in her mother's arms. She twisted, leaning into the embrace, to find a majestic barred owl at her back. Its eyes shown like obsidian, spiraling her into their depths. She breathed in its sultry breath. The owl bent its head to touch her forehead. The dense feathers felt as soft as milkweed fluff against her fevered skin.

"I will always be right here," the owl murmured—or thought—into Avy's mind. "Now get up. Be strong. You are meant to fly." Powerful wings unfurled to span across the sky. They enveloped her in a brief embrace, then the owl lifted from the bark mound to wing into the forest.

———— ◆ ————

The room was dark when Avy woke from the dream, feeling both refreshed and comforted. She checked her watch and saw it was past 7:00. She drew herself up from the bed and left the room to see what she could find for dinner. She felt, surprisingly, as though she could face whatever lay before her with her father. But tomorrow she had to continue her trip to Albany and the interview.

Chapter 9

"Leave a message at the beep. Your call will be returned at our earliest convenience." She ended the call. She had already left two messages for her sister before setting out for her interview in New York. A third would not magically result in a return call. Auralei could be counted on to do *everything* at her convenience—if at all. She wondered how her sister could run a business when she didn't answer the phone or return calls.

After eloping right out of high school, Auralei and her husband, Leandro Diaz, had headed east, and both families eventually lost touch with them, and with each other. But a few years later, there she was—posing provocatively in an American Eagle ad in Avy's *Seventeen* magazine. Then it was nearly six years before she saw or heard anything from her sister. She had leafed through an old *Vogue* magazine in the nurses' lounge. There, she spotted Auralei's photo and name in an article touting the up-and-coming young fashion designers of New York. Her sister's designs were being produced under the label "Aura" for one of the top fashion houses in Manhattan. Avy had used a hospital library computer to look it up on Yahoo and chanced sending a letter to Auralei at that address. Her sister's voice on the phone a week later took her by surprise. They had managed to keep in touch sporadically for a couple of years, but now she wondered if Auralei was still in New York. Had her success taken her to Milan or Paris?

Approaching Michigan's capital on her drive east, Avy made her decision. Instead of taking the slim chance she could meet up with Auralei in Manhattan, she'd head straight through Ontario on her way to Albany. It would cut off an hour and a half of driving and she could focus on the interview instead of how she might enlist her sister's help in managing their father. She exited Interstate 96 onto I-69 and merged into the heavy traffic heading to work in Lansing.

She sped up, feeling the tempo of purpose beating in her chest, along with the classic rock station WMMQ. Moving with energy into the stream of the powerful people—the people who ignored the limits to make the opportunities they needed to climb higher— she told herself that this was where she belonged. The people who earned respect as they earned their high salaries were her people. Her hands gripped the wheel as she maneuvered around the stubborn few who obeyed the speed limit. She felt a half smile creep up one cheek as she searched the faces in the cars she passed, pitying them for their lack of ambition. Her ribs expanded to take in a deep, purposeful breath. She rolled her shoulders and jutted out her chin with self-satisfaction. The year 2000 beckoned to her with promise, and she was ready.

Three hours later, she had crossed into Canada, navigated through Sarnia and found herself cruising along on Highway 401 past one snow-dusted field after another. Barns stood lonely under the threatening skies and even the farmhouses seemed shut up for the encroaching winter. The only signs of life were the creaking windmills turning in the stiff wind that buffeted the car. Her wrists ached from keeping it on the road.

With relief, she saw a sign for the Woodstock Travel Plaza. A shot of caffeine would reenergize her and a Tim Hortons glazed doughnut would quiet her growling stomach. Later, she reasoned, she could find a more healthful choice for dinner. She exited into the parking lot and shut down the engine. Rolling her head to release her taut neck muscles, she stretched her arms over her head and pushed against the ceiling, then opened the door. As she slipped one foot out, the wind slammed the door back into her outstretched leg.

"Kudzu!"

She rubbed stiff fingers over her bruised shin and braced her knee against the door. Now she could hear how strongly the wind screamed across the lot. She snatched up her purse and hurried to the double door of the travel plaza and the promise of warmth.

<hr />

She swiped the napkin across her lips, removing the last crumbs of her doughnut, and hoisted herself out of the booth on stiff legs. As she turned to leave, she bounced off the belly of a beefy truck driver in a Toronto Maple Leafs sweatshirt, sloshing his coffee across his chest.

"Whoa! Watch yourself there, young lady," he boomed. "No need to be in such a rush to get back out there." He pointed out the window, then rubbed at the wet stain with his sleeve.

"I'm so sorry!" she exclaimed, mentally correcting the hockey team's grammar—leaves, not leafs—and noting through the plaza window that snow had begun to swirl down in earnest. "Can I buy you another coffee?"

"Only if you'll get yourself one and keep me company with it."

Her ears buzzed a warning, but she felt she ought to do something to make up for her clumsiness, so she agreed. Besides, she was glad to have an excuse to remain out of the wind a little longer.

She returned to the booth she had just vacated, carrying two coffees and a forty-pack of Timbits. She set them down before the trucker and slid back into the booth across from him. "So, you're a Maple Leafs fan," she said.

"Best ice hockey you'll ever watch!" His damp chest puffed out. "You're not a Canadiens fan, I hope," he added with a threatening growl, scowling at her across the booth.

"I don't know much at all about hockey so, no, not a fan."

He grinned. "So you never heard of Ace Bailey, then."

"Nope."

"Well, he's a legend! He took the Maple Leafs to the Stanley Cup in '32. His jersey, number 6, is still hanging from the rafters at the Scotiabank Arena."

"That was before my time."

"Mine too—just. But I got to meet him when I was eight years old, ten years after his retirement. He was a fine man, positive and optimistic after his awful injury. I've been a fan of his and the Leafs ever since."

"Well, I'm headed for Albany, New York. Any hockey teams there?"

He rubbed his chin with a sausage of a thumb, leaving a smear of powdered sugar in its wake. "None that's worth a damn. There's the Buffalo Sabres just over the border, but they're unpredictable and volatile—which is not necessarily a bad thing on the ice, but they take it off the ice, too. You could go with the New York Rangers, but they've been in a terrible slump. If you want to root for a winning team, like I said, the Maple Leafs."

"I'll give it some thought," Avy said, high-fiving him across the table, "but right now, I'd better get back on the road before this snow gets any worse."

"Let me give you some advice, then. You're crossing over at Buffalo? Try to follow behind a big rig when you head out. We're a little slower, but we make a path through the snow that makes it easier for you little guys. You could follow my lights as far as the next exit, but from there I'm heading north."

"That's good advice. Thanks. But it doesn't look too bad yet. I'll take my chances."

"Okay, doll. Thanks for the coffee and the bits!"

The dusting of snow was still that, just flurries eddying across the road. Like two nights ago when she found herself driving in Michigan instead of Indiana. Well, she was back on track now, heading for Albany and that corner office that she deserved. The car, a little the worse for having collided with a giant metal cross, still drove fine, although she suspected she'd need to get the wheels realigned. They were pulling, a bit to the right, just as her concerns kept pulling her from her goal back to her father.

She could see a big rig bearing down on her in the rearview mirror. She'd never gotten that guy's name, she realized. But then she'd never see him again. Her internal warning system must have been out of whack, too. He was nice. Especially after she spilled coffee all over his precious Leafs sweatshirt.

The unmistakable thrumming of rumble strips brought her attention back to the road ahead. She jerked the wheel to the left, just missing the sign for the next rest stop, and the snow sent the Focus skidding across the lane and into a 360 spin. She pulled out of it, all senses alert now, miraculously heading in the right direction, and continued down the highway. The truck was gaining behind her, lights flashing and horn blasting. Shaken, she signaled to turn off into the rest area, slowed, and found a parking spot away from the other cars. She felt cold sweat snaking down her back and her heart racing in her chest. She turned her head away as a car crept past her, and she saw that the eighteen-wheeler had pulled into the rest stop too and was drawing up beside her—no matter that it was "car parking only."

"Chicory" she mumbled in embarrassment, as the familiar face of her coffee companion appeared in the truck's window.

"Are you okay?" he yelled, jumping down from his truck.

Chagrined, she turned to face him, and rolled down the passenger window. He rested his hands on the frame, his eyes searching hers.

"I didn't notice how badly my wheels were out of alignment. I overreacted when I hit the rumble strips. Whew! Maybe it was all that coffee we drank at Tim Hortons. Thanks for checking on me, but I'm okay now. I'll take your advice, slow down, and follow behind a truck for now. You're about to turn off, right?"

"Yeah, I unload in Kitchener. Promise me you'll take it easy, okay? This stretch gets much more snow than people expect—lake effect squalls that dump a lot fast." He straightened, patting the window frame twice. He looked reassured that she seemed to take his warning to heart.

"I promise. My name's Avy, by the way. What's yours? I like to know the names of my guardian angels."

He slapped his gloved hand back down on the edge of the window frame.

"Oh, that's rich!" he laughed. "It's Gabe! Short for Gabriel!"

Chapter 10

In the morning, Avy woke to her alarm, well rested in her bed at the Washington Park Inn, where the hospital had secured a room for her. She had arrived too late the night before to take in the scenery, so she carried her breakfast outside to sit on the porch and watch the sun rise over the park. The air was crisp, but she was warmed by her coffee and a wool throw that had been draped invitingly across the rocker. She had three hours before her interview.

Most of the foliage had long ago dropped from the trees, but a stand of red oaks in the park still held on to their burnt-sienna leaves, reluctantly letting go one at a time. Gray squirrels leapt among them, searching the light snow for any missed acorns to add to their winter cache.

A chipmunk chittered from the dry rhododendrons beneath the edge of the porch, and she became aware of other sounds—jays scolding from the branches above, the rustling of dry leaves blowing across the walk, footsteps of joggers passing by, and the rush of tires as people headed to work.

It was time to review her notes and prepare for the interview. This was her second chance and there was no kissing Judas around

to betray her this time. It was up to her alone to win this role. She
headed back indoors.

⸻ ◆ ⸻

A few hours later, Avy sat in the outer office of the administrative suite.
She wore the same dove-gray suit and raven heels, but this time she
had exchanged the red blouse for a new, delicate rose one; her lips glistened with a subtle whipped berry shade. She had swept her hair into a
tight chignon fastened with an opalescent pin she had bought in a vintage shop back in Denver. She carried her black leather briefcase with
a second copy of her résumé, her research notes on the hospital, the job
description for the chief nursing officer, and a brown suede notebook
with a list of questions. She had memorized them, but would make a
show of noting the responses with a shiny, black Montblanc pen. She
felt as ready as she could be to impress the interview team.

Yet a nagging voice in her head clamored in the stillness of the
room, reminding her of the havoc that could be occurring back
in Berndtbridge with her father. Somehow, she determined, she
would enlist the aid of her siblings to put order to the situation back
home. A second voice taunted her with her recent failure at Saint
Stephen's, but now everything was up to her and how she presented
herself to the woman stepping through the doorway of the Human
Resources waiting area. Avy silenced the internal monologues and
stood briskly. With her best expression of confidence, she reached
to take the woman's outstretched hand.

"Aviana? I'm Dorothy Henderson, chief operations officer for
Saint Catherine's."

"I'm pleased to meet you, Ms. Henderson." She let go of the
cool hand that had gripped hers firmly, hopeful that her own grip
had indicated enthusiasm.

"We're so pleased that you would make this long trip to meet with us." The woman ushered her through a polished cherry doorway and into a softly lit hallway hung with soothing oil paintings of forested mountains under Aegean-blue skies. "I hope your stay at the Inn was restful?"

"It was lovely. Thank you for arranging it." Her guide smiled, and Avy resumed as they continued down the hallway, "I'm thrilled to be considered for this opportunity and I'm looking forward to learning more about the facility. You're doing wonderful work here from what I understand."

They reached a glassed conference room and her escort paused before the door.

"Yes, we're quite proud of our reputation and we're serious about the people we ask to join us. Let me introduce you to the team." She held open the heavy glass door for Avy to precede her into the brightly lit room.

<hr />

When Avy passed back through the door an hour later, her eyes were alight with confidence. She knew she had responded well to their questions, and their faces had reflected satisfaction.

Ms. Henderson led her on a tour of the hospital, including all of the units where nurses scurried in their tasks. Avy made note of their expressions as they rounded corners in her path or spoke with anxious patients and family members. While they were clearly busy, their demeanor showed compassion, care, even pleasure in their work. As she glanced into rooms that they passed, she noted equipment that was up-to-date, med-carts that were orderly and locked, and staff documenting findings on mobile computer stands. All seemed to be running as it should in a well-staffed and

-resourced medical facility. She would fit right in. Assuming—
and she must not allow herself to assume again—that she was the
candidate that they chose. Yet she knew she had done well in the
interview. It was hard not to assume that she would soon direct this
nursing department, but she damped down her expectations; she
would allow herself only a small dollop of hope.

"I'm truly impressed with Saint Catherine's," she offered
in parting, and to make the point, listed several things that had
impressed her.

"It's been a pleasure getting to know you, Aviana," her escort
responded. "You can expect that we'll be in touch within ten days.
Have a safe trip back."

With another firm handshake and bright smile, Avy answered,
"I'll be waiting eagerly to hear from you."

Avy risked a friendly parting wave as the revolving door took
Ms. Henderson back into the facility. Once she'd gotten things settled for her father, she could get back to her own life—and she felt
that Saint Catherine's would be a great place to move forward with
it. She had hoped for a hint, but she had plenty of other things to
keep her busy and her mind occupied while she waited for the call.
She turned from the building and entered the parking lot.

She found her Focus and tried Auralei's number again with no
success. Even that didn't wipe the smile from her face, and she set
the GPS for her sister's last known address in the Inwood neighborhood of Manhattan. As she headed toward the highway, her body
warned her of two things simultaneously: she hadn't eaten since
early that morning, and she really needed to pee. She swerved into
the lot of Au Bon Pain just before the highway entrance.

Chapter 11

Avy crossed over the Tappan Zee Bridge and headed south toward Manhattan. She wondered again if she was on a wild goose chase, if she'd be able to locate Auralei, but she had to try. Her sister's last address was on Vermilyea Avenue in Inwood. Her GPS brought her past food venders, a barber shop, a *lavandería*, and a *mercado* whose wares burgeoned onto the sidewalk. A sign welcomed her to the neighborhood of Little Dominican Republic.

She rolled her window down a few inches despite the chill, to take in the lively music spilling down from apartment windows like raindrops. She nearly missed hearing the GPS announce she had reached her destination, the entrance to a five-story brownstone. She parked at the curb under a leafless tree, like others that lined the avenue. Skirting a teenager practicing kickflips on his skateboard, she took the four steps up to the door and entered the lobby. The apartment numbers lined up by the intercom but were without names. She pushed the number that she hoped she recalled for the Diaz apartment and held her breath. A click and a male voice crackled, "Qué?"

"Lee? Is that you?"

"No, te equivocaste de apartamento."

"Leandro?" She managed to get it out before the intercom went silent.

"Sí, está Leandro." The voice switched to English. "Who wants to know?"

"It's Avy. Auralei's sister. Is she home?"

The buzzer sounded to let her into the apartment building and she pulled the lobby door open. The spicy scent surrounding her combined cinnamon, chili pepper, garlic, and other ingredients she didn't recognize. Her stomach rumbled.

Two flights up, she heard a door open and Leandro called out, "Up here!"

She rounded the landing and spotted him in the doorway. Although he was thirteen years older than when she'd last seen him leaning against his locker, his boyish high school charm had grown into a handsome masculinity.

"Avy. You've grown up. I wouldn't have recognized you. Of course, we didn't really see much of each other back then anyway." He opened wide the apartment door and she stepped in.

"You look great, too. I'm so glad you're still living here. I've been leaving messages for Auralei, but she's not returning my calls. Is she home?" She craned her neck hoping to see her sister emerging from a bedroom.

"She's not here. But she might be 'home.'"

Her brow furrowed as she waited for him to explain.

"She quit the big firm she was with a year ago and went into business for herself as 'Golden Aura.'" His mouth and eyes went wide, and he waggled his fingers in the air. "I guess plain old 'Aura' wasn't good enough. She's got an artist's loft down in the garment district. She does all her design work and sales from there, and lives in an apartment at the back."

"But—"

"We're not together anymore. Separated, but I expect to receive divorce papers any day." He spoke matter-of-factly, but turned away from her to pick up an empty Corona bottle from the floor. "She's a hot young designer now," he added, throwing the bottle into the overflowing trash can. "And that image doesn't go well with a high school soccer coach." His mouth twisted up tightly on one side and his nostrils flared as he flipped his hands over and shrugged.

"I shouldn't be surprised," Avy said, "but I had no idea. I'm sorry, Lee—Leandro."

"Yeah, me too. But this is who I am, and I like it. She didn't."

She scanned the apartment again and noticed what she hadn't a moment ago. She was standing in a man cave with no sign of a feminine presence. She felt an unlikely kinship with Leandro— betrayed by someone he trusted.

"Auralei always was a narcissistic little b—butterbur," Avy blurted.

"A narcissistic what?" Leandro grinned. "Oh, never mind. If it means she thought only of herself, I can't argue. Listen, I can give you the address if you really want to see her."

"Yes, please. Much as I dread it, I really do need to get in touch with her. Does she have a new phone number along with a new address?"

His back slumped away from her as he crouched at the coffee table and wrote out the information. "She has a second phone now for her business, but she still keeps the old number for calls that she chooses to screen. That may be why she didn't return your call. She's all professional now and probably didn't want to be reminded of her old life. I only left her a message on that number once since she left, and she didn't call me back either." He rose, turning back to her, with the scrap of paper. She pocketed it.

"Well, this is a bit awkward," he said, "but I need to get to school for P.E. classes, so I'm gonna have to show you out."

"Yeah, I won't keep you. Listen, I apologize for my sister."

"No need. It was weird—but nice—seeing you, Avy, after all this time. I never expected to see any of Auralei's people again." He reached behind her and opened the door. It let off a sound like Chewbacca communicating with Han Solo. "Ten una buena vida—Have a good life."

"You too." They hugged awkwardly and she turned to the stairs. She heard the apartment door shut behind her as she reached the first landing.

"Ten una buena vida. That's the plan."

Avy parked her car in an exorbitantly expensive lot a few blocks from Auralei's studio on 37th Street in the Garment District. If her sister wasn't there, she figured she could easily make it back within a half-hour, avoiding the higher rate. And if Auralei *was* there, well, it might be worth the price. If she could control her judgmental attitude. Even so, she could probably rescue her car before the clock ticked over into the day rate. Still in her interview suit, she merged with the fashionable New York crowd pushing through each other as they rushed to their next meeting or business lunch. Carried along in the current of bodies, she just managed to extract herself from the mob in time and slip into the doorway of her sister's building. She was glad there was no doorman there to run interference.

She approached the listing of offices and apartments and found the name "Golden Aura."

"Here we go."

Heading for the elevator, she took a deep breath, wishing she had an idea of how to approach her unapproachable sister. On the top floor, she stepped from the elevator and came face-to-face with the door to Auralei's atelier.

Beyond the frosted glass door, two figures swept by like ghosts. And the ghostly voice that seeped through the glass was—yet was not quite—recognizable as that of Auralei. She was about to knock when the door swung open from inside the studio.

"Return a week from today, and your alterations will be complete. We'll have a final fitting then to ensure that everything is to your satisfaction."

"I'm sure it will be. You've never let me down, Aura."

As the customer stepped toward the elevator, Auralei's eyes swept over the newcomer standing in wait.

"Ah, I don't believe that I scheduled another appointment, but I'm happy to meet a new client."

She smiled coolly, looking Avy up and down, and beckoned her inside with a regal sweep of her hand. Auralei wore a black silk dress split diagonally up the front to reveal her svelte legs. A large black gemstone set in gold hung from a chain between the folds of her deep surplice neckline. Something from her memory arrested Avy as she was about to step across the threshold. Her pupils narrowed as she gazed into the lambent interior of the stone. It was disturbingly familiar somehow.

A small impatient cough released her from the seduction of the gem, and she slid past Auralei into the luminous room. She realized that her sister didn't recognize her—the ugly duckling, in the presence of the glorious swan again.

She took a moment to absorb the showroom before having to face her sister. Perhaps it was the result of the sunlight pouring through the floor-to-ceiling windows, but Avy could swear there really *was* an aura to the garments draped on faceless mannequins and the shimmering fabrics lined up on a polished oak rack. Even the golden oak flooring shone. An alluring scent emanated from a room diffuser centered in a glass bowl of yellow crystals. Shining like captured sunbeams, they drew attention to the bottles of Golden Aura perfume and boxed essential oils arranged beside the bowl. Vapor rose from the diffuser into the air to lap at the framed diploma from the Fashion Institute of Technology on the wall above. She was surprised that her sister had returned to school, even if it was for a flimsy degree in fashion design.

Behind her, the door whispered shut, and she turned. Auralei was speaking. "You're wanting a whole new look, I imagine. That washed out shade of gray is very much last year. And paired with that pink blouse—is that a faux silk blend? Altogether, it says you're going to an interview for a boring job at the most mundane sort of establishment. But I can fix that."

"Auralei."

Her sister's eyes snapped up from perusing Avy's outfit and met hers.

"Oh!" Auralei's mouth shut and she took a step back, pivoted, walked to the desk, and leaned her weight on it. Avy remained where she was. Auralei took two deep breaths that seemed to strain her willowy body. She straightened to her full height—balancing on four-inch stilettos—and swung around to face her sister. Her face arranged itself into a thin smile.

"How did you know where to find me?"

"I went to your old address. Leandro told me."

"Ah. So he was home, not working up a sweat running around with all those oversexed, underskilled teenagers he calls athletes."

"I seem to recall that you were rather enamored of a certain oversexed athlete yourself once."

"Yes. Well, I grew up. Look around you. Look what I've accomplished." Her right arm swept the room in a balletic arabesque.

"I'm impressed," Avy said, lifting an eyebrow and a shoulder in unison. "You've certainly made something for yourself—Aura. I must say, that's a more sophisticated name than Auralei." Her older sister held herself at her full height, arms crossed over her flat chest as if guarding the perimeter of her body, keeping her distance from the lesser being that dared to enter her space. She said nothing—there was no need. Avy could feel the disdain pouring from her sister's eyes, condescension leaking from her carefully concealed pores. But the years of jealousy that Avy thought she had banished away to a little corner of her soul had taken over her voice. She couldn't stop herself.

"Did you change your name legally or is it just a stage name? This is an act, isn't it? Or is it? You've always been a bit of a snob, looking down on everyone else." A voice in her head warned that she was sabotaging herself, blowing her chance to reconnect and engage her sister's help, but the bitterness continued to pour out, escaping from that hard pit in her soul. The strain of maintaining a confident aspect for her interview that morning had taken its toll. Her carefully crafted image had disintegrated and the fettered anxiety broken loose in the face of her polished sister's scorn.

"You were so eager to be free of our family, like you were too good for us. You didn't consider anyone but yourself, and you left me to manage on my own, to fend for myself while you were off doing your own thing." The accusation echoed hollowly in her memory. It was the same thing Jared had said about her!

She choked back the remaining unspoken reproaches, tasting bile in her throat. Auralei remained poised as a statue with a Mona Lisa lift to her lips that twisted Avy's stomach.

"Are you finished?"

Humiliation gripped her. Her hand flew to her mouth as she felt her stomach cramping. Her knees trembled and threatened to buckle. Darkness crept into the corners of her vision and she could only sense a hand now gripping her elbow. "Avy? Avy!" Her sister's voice cut through the darkness and demanded, "Don't you dare!" She was dragged through a doorway and dumped onto the floor in front of a toilet bowl. The door slammed shut behind her. First the croissant, and then the delightful breakfast she had enjoyed hours ago left her body, and then for an interminable time she dry-heaved.

Finally, she raised her head from the cool porcelain and flushed the stink away. She rose shakily and pivoted to sit on the lid. All was quiet on the other side of the bathroom door. She reached for a plush washcloth, wet it in the stream of cold water in the sink and held it to her forehead.

She had bungled this badly, she realized. She couldn't hear any sound of voices or movement and hoped no clients had entered the shop while she'd been throwing up behind the apartment door. Stealthily, she cracked open the door of the bathroom. Now she could hear a voice from beyond the wall, in the showroom. She picked up her shoes, which had fallen off at some point in her mortifying stumble from her sister's airy shop, and tiptoed, stocking-footed, from the bathroom into the studio apartment.

She sized up the mini fridge, the toaster oven, and the Mr. Coffee plugged in by the miniature kitchen sink. Several white plates and mugs rested in the bamboo dish rack. She peeked into a tantalizingly open cabinet. The darkness inside revealed a box of herbal tea, a jar of mixed nuts, and an unopened bottle of Rose's Mojito mix. She would have loved some of that herbal tea to settle her stomach, but she didn't dare.

She held herself steady on the edge of the counter and focused on the rest of the small living space. Under a window, a rumpled daybed stood. Only one other window allowed a bit of sunlight in from the east, bouncing off the window of a taller office building across an alley. It was not what she had expected to find behind the showroom—a humble studio apartment for the haughty Aura.

She pivoted slowly and was startled by a dressmaker's dummy, pierced with pins that held fabric in place, glistening softly in the dim light coming from the window above the bed. The dummy appeared to preside over a wall-length sewing station—cabinets of threads and sewing notions, portfolios of original patterns, and a worktable strewn with tissue, scissors, and fabric swatches. Avy skirted the headless mannequin and approached the worktable. She had never seen a sewing machine like the one before her. Four threads snaked out from oversized spools, disappearing into the machine to reappear threaded into separate needles. The sewing stool poised at the table was a saddle-shaped, ergonomically adjustable red-leather pedestal. Avy slid onto it, feeling the bones of her pelvis and spine relax into its curves. She bent to slip her shoes back on.

The door behind her clicked open and she spun around on the stool, nearly losing her balance. Auralei stood in the doorway, the warm light from the showroom pooling beneath her. Her hair glowed golden.

"Now that you're finished being sick, do you want to tell me why you tracked me down here? I've got a half-hour at the most before I expect anyone else, but I've locked the showroom. My customers know to press the buzzer if the door is locked." She shut the inner door to the apartment and paraded the twelve feet across the room as if she were on a runway. Then she arranged herself on the daybed, leaning on a satin-swathed bolster pillow. She dangled one black stiletto from the toes of her right foot, the better to display the Louboutin trademark red sole.

If it was all meant to impress or intimidate her younger sister, it succeeded. Avy felt herself shrinking, just as she had as a child in Auralei's presence. Her hope for cooperation seemed ridiculous.

She felt unsteady on the stool, as if it were still turning on its axis. She braced one foot on the floor and the other on a radial support projecting over a wheel of the chair. She filled her lungs with air and straightened her shoulders.

They weren't teenagers anymore, in competition for attention. She needed to stop letting Auralei make her squirm. She could acknowledge her sister's success, but she had become successful, too. She wanted to wipe the snooty sneer off of Auralei's face. She adjusted her weight on the stool.

"Well, you were right. I *was* on a job interview. Fortunately, it was upstate, away from the snobbish elites that you cater to. They were more impressed by my professionalism and my experience than my last-year's-gray suit and sensible shoes. I'm quite confident that I'll be in their C-suite before the end of the year."

"Well, good for you," Auralei said. "If that's what you want."

Avy rushed to segue into her request. "And that's why I'm here. Before I move out east, I need to make sure Dad's got some proper support. He's losing it, Auralei. I stopped there, thinking it was for one quick overnight, but I found that he's not safe to be alone. He's drinking heavily for one thing, and behaving very erratically. I had to collect him from a holding cell at the police station! He's got multiple overdue bills that he's ignoring. I have no idea if he's taking medication properly, but he certainly isn't eating properly. I called Jared to fill him in, and I tried to reach you before I came out here. We need to do something."

"We?" Auralei stared at her, a crooked smile mirrored by an upturned eyebrow. "There is no 'we' here. I left 'we' behind years ago. I want nothing to do with him. But if you want my permission to put him in a nursing home, you've got it." Her right shoe continued to dangle, like an oak leaf refusing to fall.

"He's your father."

"Ha! He's never acted like a father to me. Yes, he paid attention to me, but not the kind I wanted. I always thought I must be adopted given how I was so irrelevant to the rest of you. I always felt like an outsider." She reached for the pendant at her chest, rubbing the stone absently. "You, at least, had a mother who doted on you, and Jared had Dad. I wasn't anybody special in that family— not even to you."

Auralei thought she was adopted? Avy had wondered the same thing about herself—anytime her father looked right through her. Except that her mother always made her feel loved. She wondered how she could have missed what her sister was feeling. She'd always thought Auralei *despised* her, but instead she was *jealous.*

Auralei's cool mask cracked before Avy's eyes. She tried to hide the tears forming with a swipe of her finger under her eyes— the same finger that now raked through her hair in defiance. "At least my art teacher thought I was something special. And she was right!" She kicked off the dangling shoe, tugged off the other, and threw it at the wall. She strode in silk-stockinged feet to her sewing station, still towering over Avy.

"This is who I am now, Avy. I'm an artist. And I'm brilliant at what I do. No one thinks I'm inconsequential here. I've made a name for myself. I'm Aura! I never want to return to the old insignificant 'Auralei.' And that's especially true when it comes to having dealings with that old bastard in Berndtbridge."

"But I envied you, Auralei." Avy rose and took a step toward her. Her sister tossed her hair, retreating with arms recrossed over her breasts.

"Well, you can go right on envying me now that I've remade myself." A bell chimed in the studio. Auralei retrieved her heels, slipped them on, and waltzed through the apartment door into the studio, ignoring her sister's presence. Avy followed, her shoes pattering on the floor, and listened at the door.

"Just drop it there, Chaz, while I sign for it."

Avy was relieved that it was a delivery, not a client. She waited, but she couldn't be sure the deliveryman had gone. It would be awkward to walk through the door and interrupt, even if it was just a delivery. And even more awkward if Auralei decided to return to the apartment and found her listening at the door. Instead, she checked out both windows hoping there was a fire escape so she could sneak away. There wasn't.

The apartment door reopened and Auralei strode toward her, the black pendant drawing Avy's eyes deeper into its center in the dim light. And suddenly she remembered. The stone had always rested against her *mother*'s breast, against the scar that ran across her throat.

"That's Mom's pendant!" Her body lunged forward as Auralei stepped back. "You stole it!" Her sister stared her down and Avy glared back.

"So what if I did? She was *my* mother, too, and I have nothing else of hers. I'm sure you grabbed whatever you could, too."

Avy's eyes fastened onto the gem. She had always loved the way it matched her mother's unusually dark, sedimentary eyes, which contrasted with her golden-blond hair. Eyes that reflected the black soil nurturing the growing things they both loved. Avy ached with renewed longing for her mother and the pendant now around her sister's neck. But it was pointless to hope that Auralei would relinquish it.

She forced herself to relax her posture. Auralei's mouth curved into a victorious smile as she, too, regained her composure and took control of her realm.

"You'll have to go now. I have an appointment arriving soon."

She hustled Avy, defeated, into the glowing showroom and reached into the glass bowl. "*I* can't help you, but here—take a crystal. It's citrine. It'll cleanse and open all your chakras and help with that self-esteem issue you've always had. And it promotes professional success. So maybe *it* can help you since you're starting that great new job you think you've got." She pressed the luminous yellow gem into Avy's hand while opening the outer door.

Auralei's exotic fragrance hung in the air of the hallway even after she had closed the door. A tall woman exited the open elevator and sidestepped her with a condescending glance. Avy slipped into the elevator, the citrine cutting into her palm, and descended.

Chapter 12

Once again, the first movement of Bach's *Concerto Number One in D Minor* broke into her sleep. As she lay in bed, she pictured her father swaying on the piano bench, his fingers tripping across the keys. For three days, since she'd returned to the house in Berndtbridge, this had been her wake-up call.

It was a tricky piece to master, but her father could still play it flawlessly. She recalled hearing the notes, when the piano was in good form, tripping from the keys in an energetic flow like a stream skipping over rocks on its way to tremble on the lip of a waterfall. Then the notes would tumble in a torrent over the edge to cascade into the whirlpool at the base of the falls, before gently meandering into a second crescendo. Unfortunately, the piano, grossly out of tune, transformed the music, which should have been soothingly lovely, into discordant, guttural gulping and glugging. A chamber orchestra composed of a cricket on violin, frog on flute, toad on cello, and bittern on bassoon.

While her father continued to subjugate both the music and the piano, she dragged herself out of bed and off to the bathroom. She pulled on the sweats from the day before and determined to continue her search for his records, to get things in order before she left. On the day the lawyer had gotten him cleared of the misdemeanors, he also recommended someone obtain Durable Power of Attorney for her father so they could make decisions in his interest. Later she would have to get him declared incompetent—which, in her opinion, he clearly was. But first, she needed to make sure he made her his DPOA. If it was up to her to ensure his safety before she left, she had to know where he stood legally. Yesterday, his study had revealed nothing in the way of legal papers, not even those she had been vaguely aware of when her mother died. Now, while he was engaged with the concerto, she decided to tackle his bedroom. She had noticed boxes on his closet shelf the other day while readying his clothes for the court appearance. That was as likely a spot as any, though she hated to snoop in his things.

She reentered his dingy bedroom, floor littered again with several days' clothes, grabbed the wooden chair from the corner, and headed for the closet. In the glare of the overhead bulb, a flimsy box that had once held a fresh ream of paper looked promising. She slid it from the shelf, dusting herself with ancient fragments of some unknown debris.

Judging the heft of the box, she thought it *might* hold documents. She jumped down from the chair and turned to the bed. After dropping it on top of the disheveled bedspread, she lifted the lid. The box held two thick leather tomes with no title or author's name. Not the papers she was hoping for.

She replaced the lid and set it aside.

The next, larger but lighter, box contained a black robe and stole with blue velvet trim and gold piping, wrapped in tissue, and a black tam shaped like a stop sign—his professorial regalia.

Zero for two.

A battered brown leather suitcase now peeked out from where the two boxes had been. She pulled it down. It was heavy enough to hold what she was searching for. Its contents shifted as she maneuvered it to the floor. Two locks were imbedded in the metal edges of the opening, but no key. She pressed against the sliders beside the locks but couldn't budge them.

This has to be it, she thought. Why else would he keep this old case locked and stashed away? She carried it across the hall and dropped it on her bed. Simultaneously, down below, the music tripped to a stop. She heard the fallboard crash as it had so often in her childhood. In a panic, she slid the suitcase under her bed unopened and raced back to her father's room. Grabbing both boxes, she leapt onto the chair and shoved them back into place, then swung the chair back into the corner and flew back across the hall into her own room. She shut the door as quietly as she could and waited.

She felt like a burglar sneaking around, rifling through his things in search of something worth stealing. Her hands were dirty with dust, but also, she thought, with taking what wasn't hers. But she reasoned that she would put it all back once she had examined it.

After a few minutes her heart and breathing slowed. She slipped to the top of the stairs. All was silent below. She descended to find the house empty and the front door wide open. "Dad?" she called. No response. "Alex?" Alex hurtled across the yard and through the open door when she called his name, but her father was nowhere to be seen. She was torn—should she go looking for him or use this time to get that suitcase open? She shut the door and headed back up the stairs with the letter opener she had unearthed from the piles of mail on the kitchen table.

She dragged the suitcase from under her bed and went to work. Now she was a lock-picker—only a misdemeanor, she thought, but she was afraid she was on a slippery slope. She was entering this new stage of her life as a petty criminal, she worried, as the locks yielded easily to the letter opener. The clasps clicked open.

A few dozen musty clothbound books met her eyes. She inhaled sharply as she recognized her mother's field notebooks from years ago. She lifted them from the case to find several shoeboxes beneath. She set the notebooks carefully in a stack on the floor and turned back to the suitcase to open the first box. The familiar aroma of leather soap brought her to tears. Her strange dream from a few nights ago came rushing back as she hugged the old hiking boots to her chest. The other box held her mother's binoculars and camera. They had disappeared from Avy's cache one day, along with the boots. She suspected her father had found them, but couldn't fathom why he would take them from her and then stash them away in a suitcase.

She slid from the side of the bed to sit on the floor, rummaged in her backpack, dug the old wool socks out, and slid her feet into them. She unlaced the boots and tried them on. They were a little roomy, but she could make them work with two pairs of socks. Her mother had been tall and strong and confident, her feet striding into each new adventure in these boots, she remembered. Until those last few months.

Her hands recalled the sensation of her mother's skin when she rubbed those tired feet. The soles were firm and calloused, even when she was sick. Her fingers had massaged and warmed them with shea butter while they retold stories of their shared adventures.

But the journals where her mother had kept field notes had disappeared after her death. Avy swept her fingers over the rough cover of the journal on top of the stack and realized her father must have hidden them away before she'd had a chance to take them.

Still seated on the floor, she wrapped herself in the old wool army blanket she found at the bottom of the suitcase. Wearing the oversized boots, she picked up a musty volume and opened it. With the title of "Kirtland's Warblers," the first few pages recorded a trip she had shared with her mother to Mio, Michigan in 1981, to write a story about efforts to help restore the Kirtland's warbler population there. She riffled the pages, the familiar handwriting causing tears to blur her vision. She wiped her eyes and set that volume behind her on the bed.

There was no title on the next one, and it differed from the others in color—navy rather than brown. When she saw the date was long before she had been allowed to join in her mother's adventures, Avy nearly laid it aside. Then she flipped the page and read the first sentence.

May 7, 1973

Now I have a diagnosis. Dr. Henry acts as though knowing that it has a name should make me feel better. He certainly does. As the words 'post-traumatic stress disorder' and its clinical acronym, PTSD, rolled off his tongue, he was already scribbling a prescription and a referral.

"Make an appointment to see me in a month for a medication review," he said, herding me out of his office. He avoided making physical contact as the door shut on me like the cover of my manila case file on his desk. The file that now contains a copy of a research article from the Journal of Psychiatric Medicine and a copy of my responses to his screening tool. He needed a tool to discover that I'm depressed, anxious, suicidal, irritable, jumpy, angry? I thought it was pretty clear.

I imagined him turning from the door and moving the six or so steps to the seat I had just vacated, sweeping the tissues from the side table into the walnut wastebasket. I sensed him tugging the Waterman pen out of his breast pocket and making notes for his own study. I was his first specimen, the first he could put the new label on.

I pushed through the glass doors of the reception area with recaptured purpose. I had a diagnosis, and I knew what I had to do before my appointment in three days with the therapist. I'm a journalist again. I ask the questions and I write the story. My readership is one, but one is enough for now.

Avy was just an infant when this journal was written. Her mother depressed? Anxious? Suicidal? Not the mother she remembered. She held the book in her lap, took three deep breaths, and turned the page.

May 10, 1973

Here's my story.

I had completed three years majoring in English at Wheaton College in Illinois when I had a vocational crisis. Not unusual for single college women facing their final year without career prospects or a potential husband. Gender equality hadn't made itself comfortable there. My grades in Creative Writing were mediocre and I was too self-conscious to teach, but I loved research and I aced all my essays.

My uncle Harley was an ornithology professor at the University of British Columbia in Vancouver. He was working on a research project to track the numbers and study the nesting pattern of the crested myna. The bird had been introduced from China early in the century, but seemed to be disappearing from Vancouver. Unfortunately, the university would not fund an assistant, but Uncle Harley offered room and board for the summer and an opportunity to explore whether I wanted to become a journalist in exchange for being his research assistant. I went.

I met Cal one day at Uncle Harley's church, St. John's Anglican, where Cal served as a seminary intern. He ran the youth ministry there, and I couldn't imagine a worse fit for such a brooding young man. His brow furrowed when Uncle Harley introduced us. His hazel eyes glanced across mine, like a pebble skipping in a pond, seeking a weak point to sink deep out of sight. Apparently, the stray lock of blond hair falling loose from above my right ear caught his attention. He began to reach toward my face, checked himself, and smoothed his own carefully trimmed black hair. Cousin Jamie, that little conniver, took advantage of Cal's discomfort and volunteered me as a chaperone for the youth group's upcoming camping trip.

Cal was endearingly out of his element trying to manage a bunch of teenagers in the wilderness away from the rules of civilization. However, my childhood camping experience and my one trip backpacking in Wyoming gave me the knowledge and relative authority to bring them all back alive. At the end of the trip, he thanked me for my help and that was the last I saw of him for two weeks.

One Sunday afternoon I went to the Nitobe Memorial Garden, a pristine Japanese haven, to spend a few peaceful hours away from cousin Jamie and to write the obligatory weekly letter home. An elderly Japanese gardener caught my eye. He scurried along, eyes to the ground, stopping only to pick up a stray leaf or to rake a few white pebbles back onto the path. Then he turned a corner out of my vision. I found a bench in the shade across the pond from the entrance. Kicking off my shoes, I crossed my legs under me and felt

*a lump roll under my right ankle. I pocketed the pebble and began
the letter, filling it with the excitement of my early work with Uncle
Harley and the possible direction of my new career aspirations.*

*I raised my head to breathe in the serenity of the place when
I saw Cal enter the garden, head down, studying a white sheet of
paper—a laminated sheet like the one supporting my stationary.
I knew he would eventually meet me if he followed the "path of
enlightenment" as instructed.*

*The gardener reappeared from behind a low building, with a
wheelbarrow and clippers. He stepped silently among the low shrubs
on the small island, snipping off young buds here, whole branches
there. I had thought the place was perfect, but I realized it was his
discerning eye that made it look that way. When he removed a small
limb, I thought, yes, I can see now why that one needed to go. I
wondered, how am I being pruned? I can feel something releasing in
me, a letting go of expectations I've taken on myself.*

*It took over twenty minutes for Cal to reach me—a very good
sign, I thought. The man is not just a serious thinker. He respects
nature and harmony. And reads directions—what a bonus!*

*He dropped on the edge of the bench, hesitantly arched his right
arm across the curved top rail and leaned toward me, as the cedars
whispered in the breeze overhead. More comfortable in this ordered
place than in the wilds, he met my eyes and asked me what I thought
of the garden. We sat there all afternoon and discussed literature,
nature, philosophy, fate, the paths our lives were taking.*

*Cal himself was struggling with a vocational crisis, wrestling
with the disparity between his call to faith-based ministry and his
affinity for logic. Rather than entering seminary as planned after
graduation, he had decided that a grounding in ancient languages
would help settle the biblical conundrums that he wrestled with.
He'd entered the Classical Languages and Literature Master's degree*

program at Grand River State University in Michigan, studying Greek and Hebrew. It was his linguistics professor who cultivated his pursuit to understand the elemental roots of the Biblical languages into a love of language itself. Cal added Latin to his lexicon and the linguistics professor as his advisor. He felt that he had embarked on a new path laid out for him—but not the one he expected. This summer internship had been his last attempt to ascertain if he should still pursue ministry and enter seminary or continue on the fascinating path of academia.

My path was also unclear, like the incident that week where a trail in the Pacific Spirit forest had faded out unexpectedly and I found myself standing ankle-deep in a bog. I could envision a rustic signpost pointing me in a new direction, but was it the right path? And would it take me to a place of sustenance? Were there others on the path to walk with or to guide? I wondered if meeting Cal was a part of this journey and if our paths might coincide.

In the following weeks, we met frequently. I introduced him to the web of unkempt meandering trails through the first-growth forests of the Pacific Spirit on the UBC grounds, so different from the manicured Nitobe Garden. In the month I had been in Vancouver, I still had not explored them all, but I was drawn, again and again, to enter that quiet unspoiled space. Cal's presence there changed it from an open-air sanctuary to a greenhouse for our relationship. It was a beautiful place. The nascent air, at the beginning of the earth, it seemed, was full of possibilities. And we began to fall in love.

In September I returned to Wheaton College to complete my degree in English, with an inkling of writing for a journal, but I'd also been exposed that previous summer to nature's expansiveness and abundance. I wanted more of that. In the woods I felt—I still feel—alive, rooted and grounded, but also wild and free. I am part of the great creative mystery of birth and growth and death and,

though it may sound silly, holy purpose. In the forest, I breathe in
the incense of heaven on earth. I'm allowed to enter the sanctuary
of the Creator of life. My new goal was to somehow remain in touch
with that and use my hard-won college degree as well.

But I also wanted more of Cal. We had shared sacred spaces and
communed together in a time beyond normal time, in wild forest and
manicured garden. And it seemed our life paths now might intersect.
Saturday mornings I woke early, immediately alert in anticipation
of his weekly call.

Avy slipped the letter opener between the pages, closed the
journal, and left the house to find her father.

Chapter 13

I'm stumped, Jared. I came downstairs this morning when he stopped playing the piano, and he was gone. The door was wide open! Alex had gotten out, too. He came running when I shouted for him, but Dad has been gone for hours."

"Geez, Avy. Calm down! He's a grown man and he's allowed to take off without notifying anyone of where he's going. We didn't keep tabs on each other the last few months I was home."

"But doesn't that seem strange? You were his favorite. He was always up in your business at the same time he left me to fend for myself."

"That's when I was younger and more pliable. He gave up a long time ago on running my life once I got the balls to tell him to shove off."

"I was hoping you'd have an idea of where I might look for him—I've tried the liquor store, the classics department at the university, and the town library, but no luck. He could be halfway to Chicago by now if he got the notion."

"Why do you even care, Avy? Give him a break. He's managed without you for ten years. Just because you showed up doesn't mean he needs you to look after him."

She winced at the sting of her brother's words, more hurtful because they were true, but there was more to it than that. The journal entry that morning had painted a picture of a man she had never known—a man who struggled with uncertainty, who could be persuaded to change his course, and who could love a free-spirited woman like her mother. She needed to find *that* man.

"I don't want to argue with you, Jared, but from what I've seen, I think he needs someone in his life right now—not necessarily me, but someone. Maybe my showing up unexpectedly after all these years has thrown off his sense of time and place, but I think he's losing it. I'm really worried." She realized she'd been winding the sticky phone cord round and round her left index finger, as she used to do when she was stressed out. She quickly unwrapped her finger and wiped the grime off onto her sweats.

"Okay. I hear you, even if I disagree. You say he took the car. He might have driven to Meijer Gardens. He took out a membership a few years ago when they opened, and he may still have it. He used to go there a lot—don't ask me why. He's never been the type to be interested in flowers."

"Thanks, Jared, I can imagine that after what I discovered today. Did you know Mom started writing a journal around the time I was a few months old? I found it this morning and read the first entry. She writes about how they met in Vancouver over a summer internship. Mom and Dad spent a lot of time together hiking in a forest and going to a Japanese garden. I know it meant a lot to Mom, so maybe he's going back in time by visiting a garden here. I'll give it a shot, but can you think of anywhere else he might go?"

A sigh sounded in her right ear as accompaniment to Jared's thoughts.

"He had one or two colleagues he used to get together with, but I don't know any names. Maybe he kept an address book? Or a Rolodex?"

"I haven't found either. I did find Mom's old address book in the junk drawer, but that wouldn't have his colleagues in it."

There was a pause as she didn't know what else to say. She stood up, leaned against the edge of the table, and stared out the window into the overgrown backyard. Her eyes rested on the broken-down tree house.

"Do you remember when Dad built you that tree house? It's still hanging in the big silver maple out back."

"Yeah. I remember. I wanted so bad to use the hammer! I must have been only four or five years old, but he showed me how to hold a nail against the board and I smacked it as hard as I could. I actually managed to hit the nail and not my thumb. Just that once. I was so proud of myself. Then he took over and pounded it in all the way. I haven't thought about that in years." His voice had mellowed. She pictured him adjusting a tuning peg on his old guitar to release the tension on the B-string. A wistful smile loosened her taut facial muscles slightly, too.

"Auralei and I weren't allowed in it, remember? It was just for you and your friends. I always felt left out, even though I was too old to need a playhouse." Then, as her teen-aged self had done when talking to Andrew on the phone, Avy carried the phone to the counter and hoisted herself up. She folded her legs in to fit the corner and cupped her other hand around the mouthpiece of the phone. "Sometimes, though, I dared to sneak up there and stretch out over the floor, just to lay claim to it."

"I wondered why it smelled like girl sometimes!"

"Oh, stop. I left no trace of my invasion, and you know it!"

Her heart warmed toward her brother and filled her voice with laughter.

"So, speaking of invasions, here's a confession for you." Jared could hardly get the words out through his own laughter. "I used to sneak my friends into your room when you and Auralei were out. We'd go through your drawers and parade in front of the mirror in your bras and panties!"

"You brat! No wonder your little friends leered at us that way!"

A car door slammed. Avy unfolded from her corner, stretching her body across the kitchen sink to peer out the window.

"He's home!" She jumped off the counter, untangling herself from the phone cord, suddenly returned to the present. "Just one quick question before he comes in. Do you know where he kept any legal papers? Like a will or financial records? Or a DPOA?"

"No, but what's a DPOA? And why do you need to know? Never mind. I'm hanging up now before he finds out you're talking to me. See ya, sis."

She set the receiver in the phone cradle, slipped off the counter, and returned it to its place on the table. She busied herself at the sink as her father walked in.

"Hi, Dad. Have you had lunch yet? I was just going to fix myself a sandwich."

"I could eat."

"Great. Where've you been? I was worried."

"You've no call to worry about me. I was just out and about." He scowled.

"Well I'm glad you're back. Alex was out and about this morning, too. It seems the door wasn't closed all the way. But he came home panting a little while ago. Now he's asleep on the couch."

Her father looked over his shoulder to see the dog spread-eagled in the corner of the couch. Without looking back to speak, he turned toward the living room, mumbling, "I think I'll join him. I could use a break from being interrogated."

"Got it. I'll leave your sandwich on the table. I'm going out for groceries. Is there anything you want me to pick up?"

He dismissed her with a backhanded wave.

———— ✦ ————

Avy returned with her hands full, lugging four paper bags of groceries, mostly nonperishables. She settled them on the kitchen table. Her father was nowhere in sight, though he'd eaten most of the sandwich she'd left. The plate lay on the table with the remaining crusts.

"Dad!" she yelled. "Can you help me put this stuff away? I don't know where you keep things."

The chair in the study scraped the floor and her father appeared, dressed in threadbare underwear, smoking a foul-smelling pipe. He dug into the closest bag and lifted out a can of Hormel, then another. He shuffled to the open refrigerator and lined them up on the top shelf before shuffling back for more. She watched, dumbfounded, as he continued to line up the canned goods in the refrigerator. She shut the fridge door behind him.

"Here are the eggs, Dad," she said, handing them to him to see what he would do. He stood for a moment, returned to the refrigerator, opened the freezer compartment, and slid them onto the ice cube tray.

"I can get the rest," she offered. He shrugged and walked to the bathroom, closing the door behind him.

Avy rescued the eggs and instead loaded the freezer with TV dinners. She put the eggs, coffee creamer, milk, cheese, and vegetables in the fridge. She retrieved the canned goods from the fridge and began opening cupboards to find space to store them. In the first, she found his dishes giving way to a bag of coffee, a box of matches, a set of measuring cups, a bag of sugar, and a roll of waxed paper. She removed them to make space to put away the dishes she'd washed that morning, still in the drainer.

She dreaded what she would find next—mousetraps in the oven?

She found the mousetraps under the sink when she put away the dish detergent. By then she had cleared away other detritus— balled-up aluminum foil, dried-up pens, a salad spinner with desiccated lettuce leaves stuck to its sides, full pill bottles expired two years prior, a set of keys from the Chevy they had from before he bought the Buick. In the two now-empty cabinets, she lined up the cereal boxes, dried fruit, canned goods, and nuts.

Holding the old pill bottles, she realized she needed to check on what might be found in the bathroom. She looked in on her father, asleep in the chair in his study, and headed upstairs.

In the medicine cabinet, the door of which she had to dislodge from its rusted metal closure, none of the meds were more recent than 1996. She dropped defeatedly onto the toilet seat and heard a clank from inside the tank. She figured the chain must have come loose from the flush thingy. With a deep sigh, she hoisted the tank cover and found an unopened bottle of Smirnoff chilling against the flush mechanism.

She replaced the cover and carried the bottle to her room.

Chapter 14

O kay, Cal," Dale said. "Do you know why Aviana has asked me here tonight?"

Dale Monfort was the lawyer Avy remembered from her father's church. Monfort had worked with him on legal matters when Avy's mother died. He didn't usually handle this kind of thing, but when Avy explained her concerns about her father's state of mind, he agreed to come over Thursday night and craft the DPOA. Cal's suspicious mien and guarded posture evidenced that he was aggrieved with her further intrusion into his life. He glared at Dale, stubbornly clenching his jaw, refusing to speak. The lawyer waited a few beats before resuming.

"This form is called a Durable Power of Attorney, a DPOA. It's intended for someone to state how they want things like finances, property, and other legal issues to be handled in case they can't express it themselves at some point. It's wise to have those things in writing and to name someone you can trust to follow those instructions on your behalf." He paused again to let Cal speak, but he remained mute.

"For example," Monfort said, "if you were to decide that Aviana should be the person to act as your Durable Power of Attorney, that means she could help you take care of those legal decisions you need to make. She can be your representative."

A deepening scowl creased her father's forehead, like the craggy face of sedimentary rock deposits formed under pressure. At his hairline, the right temporal vein began to pulse visibly. She had forgotten that vein and how, even before she knew what it was called, it was her signal to back off. To her detriment, she hadn't always heeded the signal and, of course, the lawyer was oblivious to it.

He went on. "The other form, the Durable Power of Attorney for Health Care—it's like a living will. It would give your daughter permission to make medical decisions for you. You list what you do or do not want done if you're in a condition where you can't make your own decision—for instance, if you were in a coma. Then your daughter has the right to use that information to direct what happens according to your wishes."

"But I can do all that myself!" His pent-up anger burst out. "What the hell! Why should I let her take over my life?" Her father was both outraged and puzzled and—she wondered—afraid?

Dale leaned forward to rest his right hand over her father's fist on the arm of the chair. "Calvin, I'm not saying that Aviana should take over these things right now. This stipulates that she has that authority *only* if you are unable to make these decisions for yourself." The lawyer pressed on. "I've already asked my son to do that for me and I don't plan to need his help for a long time. But it's important to plan ahead. That's all we're saying. She doesn't want to take over your life. She just wants to make sure your wishes are honored." He held her father's eyes by force of will. Cal blinked first.

"Well then, let's let *my* son do this—whatever you call it. He's smart, and he already knows my wishes. She—" He pulled his eyes away from Dale finally to glare at Avy. She guessed his look was intended to be withering, but she saw it as bewildered. "She left years ago." His nostrils flared. "She doesn't care about me. Why should I let her have control?"

"Jared is only—what—eighteen, nineteen now?" Dale countered, dragging her father's attention back. "He really isn't old enough to handle this responsibility."

"Dad," Avy said, in an attempt to placate, "in a few years, if you wish, you can change it and have Jared as your DPOA." Her father kept his focus on Dale, as if she hadn't spoken.

"I understand he's in a pretty rigorous prelaw program," Dale said. "Once he's finished that, he would be the perfect DPOA, but not yet. And Aviana's right here."

"And I was doing just fine until she showed up," her father snapped. He turned from both of them to stare out into the dark.

At least this hasn't changed, she thought. He's always gotten annoyed when his decisions are questioned.

"Dad, I'm sorry, but you're *not* doing fine. When I leave for my new job in a few weeks, I need to know that I can help you from a distance." She glanced at the attorney to see that he realized she was not planning to remain in town. "There's no one else. Besides, I'm a nurse. I know the system. What if you fell and broke your hip, or you had a stroke. I'd need to arrange help for you—get you to a hospital, work out insurance stuff, whatever." She stopped. Her father continued to ignore her. She followed his gaze to look out the window at the snow falling lazily on the denuded rhododendron.

Dale broke the awkward silence. "Listen to me, Cal. If you don't have a DPOA and you can't—for whatever reason—make an important decision for yourself, some stranger will have to make it for you."

Her father leaned in till his face was inches from Dale's. "That's what will happen if I *do* sign it, too," he whispered, loud enough for Avy to hear. "And besides, her true name should really be Gaelle— you know what it means?" He smirked. "Stranger. She pretends to be someone she's not, but I know the truth. It's hidden right in her name. That's who she really is, 'Aviana the stranger.'"

Avy felt her throat closing in a familiar ache. Her father turned his head, staring at her, commanding her attention. "There was no denying the girl was hers all right, but I was never sure that she was actually mine." Her eyes were held by his as if frozen. She couldn't believe what he was saying. He wasn't sure she was really his? What a foul, ugly thing to say!

Though the lawyer's glance lighted on Avy briefly, before flitting back to Cal, her father's eyes continued to burn into hers.

"This one here," he sneered, tossing his head in her direction, "left one day without a by-your-leave. Now she just shows up again." He held her in his sights. "See how she's trying to take over? She has no damn right!"

This is insane, Avy's brain screamed. Why was she even trying to help him? He hadn't changed at all, except for the worse. He was crazy paranoid! Living in his own world. Demented for sure.

As Dale squeezed her father's knees tightly to regain his attention, her father's hold over her broke. He returned his piercing gaze to the lawyer and gripped Dale's wrists in his skeletal fingers. The eyes of the two men locked in silence. Cal's eyes challenged Dale to acquiesce to his paranoid suspicions. She became aware of the clock ticking in the kitchen as the two men stared at each other. Then the lawyer breathed in and nodded brusquely. He swept a troubled glance at her.

"Mr. Monfort," she said, taking control of herself, "thanks for your help. But I—we—will have to just let it rest for now. Can I walk you out?" Dale stood, letting her father's grip on his wrists loosen and slide down to his hands. The lawyer held his grasp briefly and nodded in farewell. Cal sank back into his wingback, arms folded, averting his eyes again.

Avy realized it was too late to manage the man's affairs with a DPOA—he would never agree to it. And now she wasn't sure she wanted to be involved. She'd let him rely on a stranger if that's what he wanted. He was no longer competent to understand and give informed consent. He was living in his own skewed reality. One day apparently clear and pliable. The next, scared, confused and angry. And she was right there with him. Scared, confused and angry.

"I would advise that you move to petition for guardianship instead," Dale said as they walked together from the house into the bruising night. "Immediately. It can take months to get it through the bureaucracy."

"But he needs two doctors to declare him incompetent, doesn't he?"

"No. You'll need only his primary doctor to write a letter documenting his lack of ability to make informed decisions. Then bring that to me and we'll file the petition with the court. They'll appoint a guardian ad litem."

"A stranger," she said.

"Until they determine if you or another family member would be an appropriate guardian. And, just so you're aware, it doesn't have to be a family member." He glanced away as he said this, and Avy realized the attorney might believe her father's suspicions were valid.

"As much as he mistrusts me, I hate to do this to him."

"Yet it's clear you have to, Aviana, for his own good, and for your peace of mind." Monfort shook her hand and stepped into his black Lexus.

Avy watched him go, her hopes for a resolution thwarted. She turned back toward the house, stopped, and stared into the shadows where snow had intermixed with the dry leaves piled up in the corner of the porch.

She couldn't bring herself to go back inside. She'd left all this hostility behind ten years ago to fend for herself. She'd fought so hard for her freedom! And she was strong! She was tough! But, weak as he was, he was usurping that hard-won independence and pulling her back under his thumb. He was even more cruel, devious, and manipulating in his dementia than she remembered when he had his wits about him. She should just get out of here and head to Albany, she thought.

She opened the door stealthily, pulled her jacket from its hook, and left without a word to her father. Her feet carried her west to the forest retreat of her childhood. The ancient oaks leaned over her, hiding her from the stars appearing like pinpricks in the sky's black curtain. The fallen wet oak leaves padded the trail and hid the exposed roots of the trees. In the past, her heart would have lightened in this sanctuary, even under the darkened skies. The forest had always calmed her fears, awakened her to awe and wonder. Not today. Her mind churned along with her racing heart.

She hated him! And she couldn't wait months to get all this in order!

In her rush to put distance between her heart and the cold eyes and poisonous words of her father, she stumbled in the darkness over a fallen branch and fell to her knees. Pounding her fists into the muddy ground, she tore the skin of her right hand on the bark of the offending branch.

"Buckthorn! Glossy buckthorn!" She raised the cut to her mouth and saw it was caked with mud. Instead she wiped it on her ruined dress pants.

Why did I bother to dress up for that meeting? What a waste!

Avy hoisted herself to her feet one-handed, holding the injured one to her chest. She stooped to wrest the branch from the ground, scattering the year's leaf mold into her hair and down her blouse. She flung the branch overhanded into the trees. The crack as it broke across an impassive trunk startled a pair of owls, who hooted their distress to the sky. She held her bloody hand in the other, turned resolutely, and stomped back along the trail.

Her father was nowhere in sight when she crept cautiously back into the house, to nurse her wound properly. The warm water washing away the remaining mud from the deeply torn pad of her hand stung. But the water's flow across her skin also seemed to soothe her jarred nerves. She was in her element, capably caring for broken flesh.

Her wound tended and her right hand bandaged, she retreated to her room. Even rumpled, the bed was inviting, and she needed sleep. But the dilemma of how to care for a father who didn't want her help had her fidgety, her thoughts and her anger ricocheting inside her skull. The room wasn't big enough to pace in. She pulled the Smirnoff bottle from under the bed and polished it off.

Chapter 15

Next morning, Avy woke from a dream in which she wandered in a dank maze of corridors, each door leading her deeper and darker. She felt the sun on her face before she opened her eyes. Light streamed through the edge of the window blind where it twisted inward. As she scrambled for her glasses and watch, her head throbbed with a punishing hangover, reminding her of what it took to fall asleep that night. It was nearly 10 a.m. She didn't trust herself to rise.

But her body craved coffee—and aspirin. She rolled cautiously to one side and spotted the journal where it had fallen last night after the vodka had taken over. The neck of the empty bottle appeared from under the bed.

I'm sure I saw aspirin in the medicine cabinet, she thought. If I can get to it . . . She steeled herself, slipped off the side of the bed to her knees, and crawled. By the time she'd dragged herself to the bathroom, the call to pee overcame the quest for aspirin's relief, and she sat, head in hands, on the toilet seat. She could reach the medicine cabinet from there, and the effort to open it knifed through her brain like shards of glass. But the aspirin was right where she recalled. She squinted at the expiration date to see that it, too, had expired. She dry-swallowed four instead of two and rested her head against the edge of the sink. Finally, she managed to weave back into the bedroom and slide carefully back into bed.

When she woke again, the headache was a dull memory. She blinked, blurry-eyed, at the ceiling, felt for her glasses on the table, and wedged them over her ears and her stuffy nose.

She was proud to have accomplished that one thing. She tested her addled body by turning her head. The room came into focus. She shifted slowly to one side and felt no urge to vomit. There on the floor lay the journal, if only she could reach it. One leg snaking out backward from under the sheet for balance, she stretched out her left arm and caught hold of the book's spine. Exhausted, she remained flopped sideways across the bed, until the renewed ache in her head forced her to swivel back onto her pillow, clutching the journal to her belly.

I think that's enough for today, she thought.

But her curiosity urged her to make one more monumental effort. She lifted her torso on two wobbly arms and pushed her palms into the mattress. Her sluggish hips dragged against the sheets until her rear was stopped by the pillow and she leaned back against the headboard. The journal fell open on her lap.

Doors opened quickly that following summer. In May, I graduated and received my acceptance into the Journalism graduate program at GRSU. Cal took a teaching assistant position there, teaching Greek and Latin for his mentor while he worked on his PhD dissertation. We leapt headlong into marriage on July 20, 1969, the day men first landed on the moon.

Cal was not anxious to start a family, and I agreed. My grad school studies engrossed me and I was anxious to start my own career. I began submitting small pieces to the local paper as class assignments. Only one was accepted—a story on the activist who handcuffed herself to the wrecking ball slated to begin demolition that day on the old City Hall downtown.

I just now realized how hard it must have been for Cal to jump into fatherhood so unprepared and fearful.

"I didn't have a very good role model," I recall him saying. "My father was an alcoholic. During the day he put on a good face for work, but before he got home at night, he'd stop in the bar. He was a mean drunk, and that's what I got to see. He saved his good side for his customers." Cal's father had died, falling off a barstool during a heart attack, a few years before we met. The man would always be a mystery to me.

"I'm just not sure I know how to be a good father," he told me.

Avy could attest to the fact that he sure didn't make a good father. But still, she was glad that he'd changed his mind. Her mother had made up for his bungling.

Nothing in those first years of our marriage is relevant to what happened. I don't know why I'm going into such detail. My therapist would probably say I was avoiding the important issue. Or she might say that whatever I felt was necessary to write down must have some importance to me. I don't know how else to come to it, though. I'm a journalist. These background facts seem necessary to record. So:

We both settled into our work. I gained a good reputation as a freelancer, then landed a position writing for the travel section of the paper. I'd never been out of North America, and the promise of travel thrilled me. Because I had no children and Cal was focused on his teaching and the dissertation, I was free to take juicy assignments abroad. I always managed to work a feature of each unique environment into the story.

Cal was the one who initiated the trip to the Netherlands. His mentor had invited him to present a paper—a shortened form of his dissertation—at a three-day conference at the Vrije Universiteit in Amsterdam. I convinced my editor that a feature on the Netherlands would have great appeal to the large Dutch population in our area.

"I can write a story tying the U.S. flower market to suppliers in the Netherlands. Maybe hand-deliver an order to the Aalsmeer auction and then track it through the bidding, packing, and shipping to the states," I pitched him. I envisioned a vibrant photograph of the Aalsmeer flower market on the front page of the travel section. And I could do a number of side bars: the Anne Frank house in Amsterdam, the porcelain factory in Delft. If he wanted a personal touch, I could try to track down some of Mom's relatives in Groningen who might still run a dairy farm.

I wrote the story, and it was more than I had promised. What I didn't write about was my repulsion at the side of Amsterdam that people like me, the travel writers, avoided mentioning. The drugs. The homelessness. The prostitutes posing in their store windows like mannequins. And coming upon Cal as I stepped off the bus, exhausted from a day in Aalsmeer and Delft. Cal, drunk with his new colleagues in a sidewalk bar, was groping the thigh of a teasing blond waitress.

So maybe it wasn't just the dementia, Avy thought. Had he always been a letch? Is that what Auralei was implying when she claimed that he gave her attention, but not the kind she wanted? He'd never been like that with her.

Disgusted, she lay back against the pillows, curled her body protectively over her mother's journal, and wondered what she had gotten herself into.

Chapter 16

Joplin's jaunty tune pierced Avy's sleep-fogged brain.

Her limbs flung out in the classic startle reflex, knocking the journal from her chest. She cried out with pain as her neck snapped out of its cramped position.

Fumbling for the phone on the bedside table, she fell out of bed to her knees, hitting her forehead on the corner of the table and sending the phone tumbling to the floor. It plinked out the theme from *The Sting* once more before she could grab it and flip it open. She pressed her right hand to her bleeding forehead and held the phone to the opposite ear.

"Hello?" she croaked.

"Aviana?" Avy recognized the voice that paused on the question. She cleared her throat and hoped her brain would follow suit.

"This is she." She attempted to inflect into the statement a brightness she didn't feel. She opened her left eye a slit to discover double images of the journal sliding clockwise across the floor while her body spun counterclockwise in sync. Her stomach kept its own pace, but lagged behind. She snapped her eye shut, but stars now orbited behind her lid. The voice on the phone resumed.

"Aviana, this is Dorothy Henderson at Saint Catherine's in Albany. Is this a good time to talk?"

"Yes, of course," she lied. "I'm delighted to hear from you."

"And I'm pleased to be bringing you this news. We're offering you the position of CNO at Saint Catherine's. We think you'll be a wonderful part of the team here. I expect you'll need some time to consider our offer, but we look forward to a positive response."

She could barely hear the voice over the ringing in her ears, but she understood she'd just been offered the position she craved.

"That's wonderful news, Ms. Henderson." Her stomach had caught up with her spinning body and clamored to be emptied. She groped for the wastebasket and clutched it to her chest.

"I'll need a little time to take care of some family business," she managed as brightly as possible, "but I can give you a positive response now. I'm delighted to accept the offer." She covered the phone to stifle an insistent belch, then continued. "I felt, too, that Saint Catherine's was exactly the kind of health facility in which I hoped to serve." Saliva gathered in her mouth.

"That's marvelous, Aviana. Please call me Dorothy. Why don't you get back to us at the first of the week and we can talk about your onboarding schedule."

She wondered if she'd heard that right. Onboarding? "That sounds perfect, Dorothy. I'll call you on Monday. Thank you so much for this opportunity."

"Until then. Enjoy your weekend."

The phone went dead as she heaved the meager contents of her gut into the wastebasket and passed out on the floor.

—◆—

Avy felt as though she were being prodded with a sharp stick. She swiped an arm back to brush it away, but now it was pummeling her shoulder. She gathered her battered limbs into a ball and kicked weakly at the perpetrator.

"Wake up, girl!"

She recognized it now as the voice of her father from long ago, calling her out of a nightmare. He shook her, pleading with her again to wake up.

"I'm awake, okay? Can you just go?" Her head ached, her brain pressing against the cavity of her protesting skull. She dared to open one eye. The room had stopped spinning, instead it seemed to recede into a shrouded stage set. She whimpered.

"It was just a bad dream. I'm here now." The hands encircled her shoulders, as if holding her together, trying to soothe.

"Let's get you back into bed now. I don't think I can lift you. Can you stand up?"

She gathered the little strength she had and lifted herself into a crouch. It was enough to waken her stomach to the need to empty itself again, but all it could produce was a series of dry heaves. Her hand found the edge of the steel bedframe and rested there, unable to do more.

"Oh dear! There's blood on your forehead." He reached out to touch her forehead and she didn't pull away. "A cold washcloth. That's what you need." She saw his knees leave the floor and his feet pivot and shuffle into the hall. It was enough movement to convince her that she, too, should attempt to rise. She was able to raise one foot to find purchase on the floor and pushed herself up and onto the bed, where she gratefully collapsed.

She realized she had a concussion. Her father had not returned with the cold washcloth, which might have helped to calm the headache.

"Dad," she called feebly. "Please, Dad. I need your help." Only silence responded.

She realized she was on her own. She couldn't rely on him to return, and she needed help. She spotted the phone on the floor, taunting her with its inaccessibility.

"Dad!" She tried to project her desperate voice into the hallway. "Daddy, please," she whimpered through tears, before passing out.

———— ◆ ————

The recurrent dream commenced.

"Daddy, please," she begged, trembling, balanced perilously between the beams in the attic. She had climbed up there, against the rules, looking for her mother's things that had been removed from her once-secret cache. He wasn't due to be home yet, but had returned early and found the rickety ladder to the attic pulled down. He glared at her through the opening.

"You came up here against my specific orders. Now you'll stay here and think about what you've done." He descended the ladder, raised it back to the ceiling and locked the trapdoor behind it. She was left in the dark, imagining spiders descending from invisible webs hanging from the rafters. Her skin crawled. She could hear faint whispers around her and pictured mice—or, worse, bats—and forced herself to stand still. She couldn't move for fear of stepping off the beam and breaking through the ceiling. How long would this punishment last?

"Please, Daddy," she whispered once more, knowing he couldn't hear her and wouldn't relent even if he did.

———— ◆ ————

A cold wetness dropped across her eyes and she yelped. Her head split into shards of pain as she flung the washcloth from her face and threw open her eyes. A blurry form stood over her, hands raised. She blinked through tears and realized it was her father.

"My phone," she mumbled. "I need my phone. Over there." She pointed roughly in the direction of the floor under the second twin bed. "And the washcloth back, please."

He leaned over and picked up her phone, tilting his head to one side. "There's no phone," he said, holding it out to her. "Do you mean your transistor radio?"

"Yes, yes! Give it to me!" She snatched it from his hand and punched in three numbers.

Her father stepped back and sat down on Auralei's old bed, watching her with curious eyes.

"Yes," she spoke into the phone. "I need you to send an ambulance to 910 Comber Row. I've got a concussion and I need to go to the ER." The robotic voice at the other end questioned her self-diagnosis.

"Of course I know it's a concussion! I'm a nurse. I hit my head. I blacked out—no, I don't know how long. I've been throwing up, and I have a splitting headache. Is that enough for you?" Her left thumb and forefinger gripped the acupressure point on the hand holding the phone. "Just make sure they know that my father will probably be the one to answer the door. He has dementia and may try to send them away. I'm upstairs." Another murmur from the phone speaker. "Thank you." She snapped the phone closed, saw her father sitting across from her, and realized he had overheard everything she'd said. She shut her eyes and let her head drop back onto the pillow.

"You can't be a nurse," his incredulous voice stated after a moment. "You're just a girl."

Chapter 17

Avy exited the cab in her father's driveway Monday morning at ten o'clock. She had passed all the tests the hospital doctors and therapists had put her through: correctly identifying how many fingers were being held up, walking a straight line, touching the therapist's finger then her own nose, counting backward by sevens, and so many more that she couldn't recall. It took more concentration than she let on—like now, keeping her balance as she ascended the two steps to the front door without the benefit of a railing.

Her father flung the door open before she had time to reach for the knob. He held in his uplifted hand the heavy bust of the Greek god Hermes that had graced his study with its deferential demeanor for as long as she could remember. Her father's own face more closely resembled that of another god—Ares, god of war. His arm trembled with the weight of his weapon and she feared that at any moment it would descend on her. She reeled back, aware of the danger of falling down the steps behind her, but her father blinked and his face morphed simultaneously into recognition, disappointment, and defeat. "You're back," he stated, and lowered the marble bust.

Not for much longer, she hoped. Relieved, she regained her equilibrium on the stoop.

"They sprang me from the hospital," she explained, indicating the blue plastic hospital bag hanging from her elbow. "May I come in?" He stepped back into the living room, turned, and shuffled off toward his study without another word.

Avy paused before following him over the threshold. She dropped the hospital bag with her few belongings on the floor and leaned both hands on either side of the kitchen doorframe, surveying the room. He had managed to survive in her absence, she noted wearily. She was glad she had bought groceries before her fall.

But in three days he had transformed the kitchen back into the chaos she had first encountered only a week ago. The refrigerator door rested unlatched against the opening. An empty liquor bottle had rolled under the table. The neatly arranged cabinets were open, their contents scattered across the countertop and stove. Used dishes sat crusting on the table.

"Giant knotweed," she murmured. She shook her head slowly and pushed off from the doorframe. "This will have to wait." It was Monday morning and Dorothy Henderson was awaiting her call. First, a hot shower to transform her back into Aviana, the capable professional Dorothy was expecting to hear from.

Exhilaration filled her after her call to Saint Catherine's. Onboarding—that strange new word for orientation—to her new position was set to start on Monday, December 6. She was back on track in her ten-year plan. By January 1, 2000 she would be sitting in that office with all its attendant rewards. She wanted to share her news with someone, but who? Only the dog showed any interest in her presence, and his was strictly selfish. A few minutes of belly rubbing and he was ready to play, not sit still and listen to her good news. Andrew, she considered. If I haven't alienated him.

Andrew seemed pleased, if not overly enthusiastic, to be invited to get together again. But it would have to be for lunch, he warned, since he was due at the police station for his shift at 7:00 p.m. He even had a place to recommend for a casual meal—the Rock River Bar and Grill.

"That sounds perfect! Does tomorrow work?" Andrew agreed to pick her up at 11:30 the next day, and she felt an old familiar flutter in her chest.

No, she thought. No fluttering! Now is not the time to be getting involved with anyone. Besides, she liked Andrew better as a buddy. And right now, that's exactly what she needed.

She found her father asleep in his study, head down at an impossible angle on his chest. With every labored intake of breath, a snore erupted. With every exhalation, another wavelet of saliva coursed down the rivulet from the corner of his mouth. Hermes— the messenger god—looked on benignly from his usual perch on the desk. She wished Hermes could help her get across the message her father needed to hear. They needed to settle some things before she left in a week and a half.

Avy stood for a while before her father, bemused by an unexpected feeling of tenderness toward him. That snoring. It recalled to her a figure pulling a chair to her bedside in the dark of a fevered night. Quietly humming a Brahms lullaby, they had placed a cold washcloth on her forehead, and had finally fallen asleep with their head dropped forward, snoring.

She didn't understand. Wasn't it her mother who had comforted her? Yet they were *his* hands, his low humming, and snoring—just as he was now. It was this man who had sat with her in her fevered state as a child haunted by nightmares, not her mother. How had she gotten it so wrong?

Chapter 18

She woke late the next day and lay in bed listening to the quietness. She saw no reason to break that peace by getting out of bed to check on her father. The journal lay on the bedside table and she drew it over to her as she scooted herself back against the headboard.

May 16

Lizzy's letter from Honduras was in the stack of mail when we returned to Berndtbridge.

"You've got to come see us in Comayagua," she urged. "I think you should do a story." The cooperatives they had helped get started were now well-organized and nearly self-sufficient. Lizzy still visited them regularly to pick up goods and deliver supplies, but both she and Joel were becoming more involved with a new initiative— supporting the efforts of the campesinos to reclaim their land. "Besides, Auralei needs to meet her namesake!"

Wait, she thought. Auralei? Mother was her sister's namesake—
Leigh becoming the -lei of Auralei—she'd always known that.
This must be a different Auralei. Of course, that must be where
she'd come up with her sister's name. But who were Lizzy and Joel?
Clearly, they were important but why had she never heard of them?
Or maybe she had and it just didn't register. Whatever. This just
made no sense.

*After Amsterdam I just needed some space away from Cal. He didn't
know what I had seen and I wasn't ready to confront him. But I
couldn't forget the sight of his familiar hand groping another woman's thigh. I didn't want that hand to touch me, yet I had allowed
it the night before I flew out. Perhaps some time with Lizzy would
give me the distance and perspective I needed to sort it out. I didn't
bother to propose the story to my editor, but I grasped the opportunity to get away and to visit Lizzy and Joel and little Auralei. I
applied for a two week leave and lied to Cal. I told him I had the
opportunity to do a story in Honduras and visit Lizzy at the same
time—maybe it would turn out to be true. He gave me a cheery
send-off the following morning, May 7.*

*May used to be my favorite month. Green appears suddenly out
of the gray-brown slush of the melting winter. All April, the gray
sky drops rain, like tears of repentance for the months of clouds
and snow, and the warm earth soaks it in. Then May arrives and
the earth awakens, as if at last offering its forgiveness to the sky
by reaching out open palms of mayapples. I can walk again in the
forest and search for signs of returning life. Rebirth and new growth
are always possible in May.*

*But in Honduras, May ushers in the rainy season. Lizzy greeted
me outside the customs area at the airport in Tegucigalpa covered
in an oversized alpaca poncho, woven with a geometric design. She*

spread her arms wide to include me under it. Her blue eyes still sparkled in spite of the tracks of crow's feet that had appeared in her weathered face. She had lost weight.

"You're exhausted," she said, and I realized I felt disoriented and emptied of everything except tears burning to be released. My little sister hugged me under the wet wool, sinewy arms wrapped around my shoulders.

Her little sister? What did that mean? She'd always thought her mother was an only child. Why had she never met this sister? She sounded like someone Avy would really like.

"So we'll head straight for home and Alejandra will fill you up with her wonderful groundnut soup and tortillas; then we'll tuck you into bed for the night. I have only a few things I need to do while you're here, and one of those is tonight." She explained that Joel wasn't along to meet me and help with my luggage because he was participating in a land reclamation.

"It's kind of like the sit-ins we used to do in Chicago." She laughed. "Joel called to say that the rain damaged most of their food items, so I need to run out there in the truck later with replacements and extra tarps."

From Tegucigalpa, Lizzy's boxy El Compadre truck climbed up the winding road to the northwest, vying with other vehicles and men on horseback. The smell of diesel fuel mixed with the scent of orchids from the roadside vendors. We topped the hills and snaked down, through the rivers of mud into a long, flat valley. There we passed a military base, like those Lizzy had written about. As dusk began to settle, we climbed higher into the mountains where the odor of burning lime couldn't smother the fresh Ocala pine breeze. Then suddenly, Lizzy piloted us down out of the forest on a road that plummeted and rose like a roller coaster into a cactus and scrub plain. Here, men in cowboy hats drew their skinny horses off the road to let us pass. Mangy dogs ran barking alongside until they were shouted back by children carrying firewood and water. Women worked the denuded hills, sowing in the downpour. By October the rain would end and the hills give up their soil to dry winds.

Their home was surrounded by a five-foot-tall brick wall, draped in pink bougainvillea. It was alive with hummingbirds in the sunset, thirsty for nectar after the drenching rain. I was surprised to see a locked wrought iron gate topped with two strands of barbed wire circled by concertina wire. It stretched across the drive and reappeared between the clumps of bougainvillea.

"In the city," she said, "there's a lot of petty theft. You don't find that out in the villages. There's not a lot worth stealing there, but here we take these precautions."

She led me through the door into a spacious, colorful gathering room, where I met her housekeeper, Alejandra, and her five-year-old son, Luis. Alejandra's soup warmed me, body and soul. Tears threatened to spill in exhaustion and relief.

"We'll catch up tomorrow after you've had a good rest." Lizzy propelled me into a bedroom and, with another hug, left me to sleep and to dream. My dreams were embellished with the birds I had seen: brilliant hummingbirds darting in the bougainvillea, raucous mountain trogons in the trees, and black vultures circling high above the house.

———— ◆ ————

Avy closed the book against the letter opener and slid it under her pillow. She ran her hands through her hair and clutched her skull, shaking her head. She blew out a deep breath. How had her mother never mentioned that she had a sister and brother-in-law? And who was this other Auralei? A niece? She just didn't get it.

The sound of choked coughing and a chair scraping across the hardwood floor downstairs brought her back to the present. She vowed to return to the journal as soon as possible and went to see what her father was up to now.

"Hey, Dad," she said, finding him standing by the front door. "Why don't we take Alex for a walk? We can talk a bit on the way."

"But I haven't had dinner yet. I always take him out after dinner."

"It's still morning, Dad. You fell asleep in your study and lost track of time."

He scowled and looked past her, searching the room for a clock.

"Here, Dad. See?" She guided him to the kitchen door and pointed to the clock on the wall, which was surprisingly accurate. "It's 11:15—in the morning. I can fix us some lunch if you're hungry."

"Why should I be hungry?" he growled. "I don't need you to feed me. Who knows what crap you'd try to foist on me. And look at this mess you've made!" He gestured at the chaos in the sink and countertops. "You can't even clean up after yourself." He stumbled back a step and, breathing hard, caught himself on the edge of the table. As if she'd pushed him, he glared at her before flopping onto the nearest chair.

"Okay. Well, how about we clean it up together. You can tell me where all this stuff on the counter goes, I'll put it away, then I'll wash the dishes and you can dry."

"Why should I do women's work? You made the mess. You clean it up." He smirked as if he'd caught her trying to pull a fast one and called her bluff.

She resisted the urge to leave him alone in his mess. Antagonizing him wouldn't help her to persuade him to accept her plan to hire a caregiver. Not only did he need to be on a schedule of eating nutritious meals, but also taking his medications, bathing, getting dressed appropriately, caring for the dog and, above all, being safe from wandering off. She also needed to make sure he got to his appointment tomorrow with Dr. Nanninga, so she could get a letter for the lawyer to move forward with the guardianship, and get his bills on automatic payment. She sighed and picked up a box of cereal to return to the same empty cupboard she had organized last week. He watched grimly, arms folded across his paunch.

"Dad. You'll be happy to know I'll be leaving in a few days. I'm moving to Albany, New York, starting a new executive position at Saint Catherine's as their new chief nursing officer."

"So, you'll disappear again, just like before."

"Isn't that what you want? You've been nothing but dismissive of me since I came. You know, *I* didn't make this mess. *You*—" She stopped abruptly. He could trigger her so easily, but she needed to maintain her self-control. Somehow, she needed him to acknowledge his need for help. She finished stacking cans and boxes on shelves and moved to put away the milk in the refrigerator. She shut the fridge door, paused, took a breath, and swung around purposefully. They stared at each other until Avy finally looked away, crossed to the table, sat down, and leaned toward her father. She would have reached for his hands but he had drawn back, his hands fisted on his chest.

"I'm worried about you, Dad."

He raised his hands in angry protest. "I told you, you don't have to worry about me. I'm perfectly able to take care of myself. Go! It can't be too soon!"

He's right, she thought. It can't be too soon, but she needed to get things set up first.

"Dad," she asked gently, "we have an appointment tomorrow with your doctor for a checkup. Can you tell me where his office is? I seem to have forgotten."

"It's right downtown where it's always been. I can go myself. You don't have to bother accompanying me to a simple checkup."

Avy knew Dr. Nanninga had moved into a large practice group near the medical center years ago, before she had left town, but her father didn't remember. And he hadn't seen the doctor in three years, according to the receptionist she had spoken to. Thankfully they had an unexpected opening. She hazarded another question to test his memory.

"You know, I haven't seen Jared lately. Where's he been?"

He batted away the question. "What's that to you? He's probably still at band practice, but he'll be home soon."

"And what about Auralei?"

"Are you an idiot?" he sneered. "Auralei ran off to Denver as you very well know. What's with all the stupid questions? This is insulting!"

"Denver, huh? Dad, Auralei is in New York. I just visited her when I was out there. *I'm* the one who was in Denver."

"No! *Auralei* went to Denver. Your mother told me she was going to visit her there—in Denver." His face reddened in anger. "And she never came back!" His face suddenly collapsed into itself. "She never came back. She found someone out there, some spic son-of-a-bitch wetback! And she never returned." Tears ran from his eyes as he pounded his gnarled fists on the table.

Avy sat in stunned silence. She wished she had a recording of that to convince Dr. Nanninga. But where had he come up with her mother running off to Colorado? Had he forgotten even that she was dead?

He scraped the chair back across the linoleum, stood, and stomped out of the kitchen. The door of his study slammed shut just as the doorbell rang. She heaved a sigh, crossed from the kitchen to the front door, and pulled it open to find Andrew standing there. He looked her up and down and a crooked smile crossed his face.

"I said it was casual, but I'm not sure the River Rock allows you to eat there in pajamas and bare feet."

"Oh, Andrew! I'm so sorry! I forgot we were having lunch! Give me five minutes and I'll be ready." Without waiting for his response, she turned and raced up the stairs.

Chapter 19

It was still dark when I woke. Loud male voices called out in a rapid-fire Spanish that I couldn't understand and I recalled Lizzy's nonchalant mention of thieves. I leapt out of bed, looking around for a weapon. I flung open my door holding—of all things—my camera bag. Alejandra was already in the common room, her dark brown eyes wide. She had just pressed the button to open the gate and was unlocking the door. "No!" I shrieked. Alejandra turned toward me and held up a hand to try to calm me.

"It's okay, Leigh. They are friends, but something is wrong." She opened the door as I ran to wake Lizzy. Auralei slept peacefully in her crib, but Lizzy's bed was empty. I watched the child only long enough to see her blanket rise and fall.

Two men stood in the common room. They gestured at me, avoiding my eyes and my questions. They just kept urging Alejandra in a language I couldn't understand, but I understood the fear that emanated from their words, scintillating in the charged air of the unfamiliar room.

"What are they saying? What's wrong?" I begged Alejandra.

"*There's been trouble at the occupation,*" *she told me.*

"*But where's Lizzy?*" *I was disoriented and confused.* "*Why isn't she here?*"

"*Please, Señora.*" *She took my hands and locked her eyes onto mine.* "*Miss Eliza did not come back. She is gone too long. They say men came with guns. I am afraid for them.*"

"*I'm going,*" *I announced, now fully awake. I still gripped my camera bag. Alejandra wrapped a poncho around my shoulders and loosened the camera from my grip.*

"*I must stay with the babies, but these men say they will take you there. These are our friends. They will take care of you.*"

I didn't look back. We rushed from the house and into a pickup truck—Lizzy's El Compadre.

I believe it was less than thirty minutes, driving in electrified silence over a narrow mountain road, when we approached a flat valley and pulled off into the brush. Beams from high-powered flashlights bobbed through a field. From between the stalks of recently harvested plantain several men emerged, moving in the direction of a small group of people gathered in a clearing to our left.

"*Madre de Dios,*" *one of the men ahead of me murmured as we picked our way in the dark over the furrows of emerging crops. Alfonso, the man supporting my right elbow as I stumbled on, crossed himself. I pushed through the fence of people. Three bodies lay on the ground, two young campesinos, probably in their teens, and one tall blond gringo—*

I knew it must be Joel.

All but their heads were covered by a blue plastic tarp. The rain washed over Joel's face, but it couldn't wash away the mess where his ears had heard the needs of these people and his eyes had looked on the injustice of their lives.

The crowd moved to my right. The yellow flashlight beam bounced eerily as four men carried in another body wrapped in a tarp. My vision waned to a blue-gray gossamer membrane. My heartbeat thudded in every cell of my body.

I fell to the muddy ground beside her. Mercifully, Lizzy's face was unmarred. Sorrow and falling rain softened the lines that had worked their way into her skin like the earth of Honduras. I gathered her into my arms and rocked her as her half-lidded eyes met mine. She looked now as she had as a child, sleepy after a bath, wrapped in a blue blanket. Mother would let me rock her to sleep. I kissed her lids and closed her eyes gently.

"Hush-a-bye. Don't you cry. Go to sleep . . ." I couldn't finish. I rocked silently as two more bodies were carried into the circle. Others moaned around me and fell to the ground beside them.

I don't know how long we stayed there, but after a while, fingers touched my shoulder and a gentle voice murmured above me.

"Señora, we must go." I looked up and saw the group moving toward the road carrying their dead in a gray dawn procession. Lizzy and I were the only ones left on the ground.

The flashlights were no longer necessary as Alfonso gathered Lizzy from my arms and lumbered over the field to the men standing with heads bowed at the trucks. I stumbled after, my legs numb, my arms aching.

<hr />

A tear spattered the page and spread over her mother's words. Avy dabbed at the stain with the hem of her shirt, then brought it to her eyes to gather the tears running down her cheeks. She took a ragged breath before she could go on.

From the window of Lizzy's pickup, I watched through the open door of the police station. The Comayagua police officer didn't even leave his chair when the men entered. He pulled forms from a drawer and lazily began to question them. But his eyes widened when Alfonso stated, "Dos Norteamericanos—Joel and Eliza Masterson."

He sprang from his oak swivel chair and loped outside. From the truck's cab, I watched the chair spin slowly to a stop, while a rapid exchange between the officer and Alfonso occurred. I sensed, through the cracked vinyl seat of the cab, the shifting of added weight in the back of the truck as the policeman dropped the wood-slat gate and climbed in to verify the identities of the bodies. Far off, black vultures rose from the river bank in the dawning east and circled slowly and silently.

"I found their passports in their belts," Alfonso said as he slid back behind the wheel. "They will keep the others here, but we must take . . ." he swallowed a sigh. "We must go to the American Embassy in Teguz with Joel and Lizzy. The officer has called the Bureau of Consular Affairs and they are waiting for us."

The smell of sweat and blood, exhaust fumes and crushed vegetation suffused the vehicle as we made our way through the empty streets and past the Parque Central and the towering Catedral de San Miguel Arcángel. Lizzy had planned to take me there that day. I could only see it as a monumental sepulcher reflecting my grief that morning. We turned southeast onto the highway to Tegucigalpa. Less than twenty-four hours ago Lizzy and I had driven north on this same road, talking over each other in our eagerness to reconnect.

Chapter 20

May 21

Only after the ambassador's aide asked did I remember Auralei. The embassy had a record of the Consular Report of Birth Abroad. With that and a photo I carried in my wallet, they would be able to rush through a passport for her. It would be ready in two days for me to pick up on my way to the airport. I would need to return to the house in Comayagua and get her. They had located Joel's brother, who asked that his body be returned on the same plane as well. Would I be willing to take possession and deliver his body to his brother? He could meet my plane in Chicago. Yes. Yes. Yes. They called the airlines, changed my flight, and arranged for the transport of Lizzy's and Joel's bodies.

Yes. Thank you. Just get me away from here. Take me home. To Cal. I can forgive him anything in a world where these horrors could happen.

I'm just writing what I remember. I wish, now, that I could remember it more clearly, but at a time like that I think you just do what has to be done. Other people tell you and you just do it.

What else can you do? Cynthia, my therapist, would remind me that numbness is one of the initial reactions to trauma.

Alfonso was so unselfish. His nephew was one of those killed that night. I didn't know until I saw a report on the news in the Tegucigalpa airport. He had declined to be interviewed about the two Americans who had been killed, but he spoke for his sister in the loss of her eldest son—sixteen-year-old Berto. Yet that day as we drove again over the road back to Comayagua, he said nothing of his own loss. Only that he would be unable to take me back to Tegucigalpa in two days. He offered me the keys to the pickup, but I refused; said he could keep it. He showed me where I could get the bus when I needed to go and dropped me at the gate of the house, where Alejandra waited.

The gate opened. It hadn't kept evil from stealing two of the greatest treasures from this house. Now I was responsible to see its last treasure, this child who had never even met me, safely to a new home. I was very, very tired.

The crying had been going on for some time when I finally woke. Auralei or Luis? I didn't even know my niece's cry. When I had returned that morning, Alejandra had already sent them both out to play in the garden. She stripped me of my muddy clothing, drew a bath, force-fed me an egg, and put me back to bed. I sank into exhausted sleep and dark nightmares.

The crying stopped abruptly as I opened the door of my room. Auralei spun around, expecting her mother, but stopped mid-dash when faced with a stranger. The wailing doubled in intensity, and this time Luis joined in. Alejandra was nowhere in sight. Both children backed away but kept me always in their sights as I stumbled through the room calling for Alejandra. She was in the kitchen, seated at the wooden table. A short dark man, flinty eyes opaque as he held me in his gaze, stood over her with one hand grasping her hair and the other holding a machete to her throat.

"Buenos dias, señora," he taunted. "You sleep late."

Alejandra's eyes warned me to stay where I was, not to come closer.

"Mi esposa here, she has been working hard since before the rooster call." He let go of her hair to tighten the rope holding her wrists. "It is not right," he said, "that she work so hard for someone else instead of for me." Finished with his work, he threw both hands wide, brandishing the machete, and laughed. "And now there is no need here. I will take her and the niño back where they belong. And you will go back where you belong."

Then he saw Auralei. She had crept up behind me and now clung to my nightgown.

I swept her up and held her. Her legs gripped my waist as if I were a pony on a carousel. She grabbed fistfuls of my hair and stared at me, finally recognizing me as the distant Auntie Leigh. I stroked her back and held her away from the man with the machete.

"Si, Señora," Alejandra begged, her almond eyes welling with tears. "Take the baby and go. It will be better for all of us."

"The niña stays," the man ordered. "She does not belong to you. She was born here. She stays here."

Fumes of cane liquor enveloped my senses as he lurched toward me. I realized that Alejandra's husband was already drunk at 10:45 in the morning. He still carried the machete, but I couldn't move. Alejandra lunged from the chair into his back. He fell to his side with Alejandra on top of him. He swung back at her with an innate deftness and the machete blade smashed into her face, leaving a gash from forehead to jaw. She fell limply onto the tiles. Still, I couldn't move.

This is all impossible. I am writing this as though I am observing what happened to a stranger, but it happened to me. Cynthia

thinks that writing this will be an emotional breakthrough of sorts.
A catharsis. I can't do the rest. I DON'T WANT TO FEEL IT
AGAIN.

The journal slipped from Avy's numb fingers silently onto
the bedspread. Her brain echoed her mother's words—this is all
impossible. Her mother had lived through a trauma completely
foreign to Avy's knowledge and experience of her. How did she
recover from that to become the serene, confident mother that she
knew? Had she known her mother at all? Her mother had a sister!
And Auralei—Avy's sister—she was actually her cousin? Her brain
buzzed trying to make sense of this information. Blood surged
through her temporal arteries like a swollen river, threatening to
burst through her ordered life. An anguished moan escaped her
throat.

Her mother had been afraid to feel it again, afraid to go on
with her writing, but did she?

Avy picked up the journal with shaking hands from where it
lay, innocuously dull and plain, swaddled in the white bedsheets.
No matter what else she might find within, the story compelled her
to go on. She cradled the book and slid with it to the floor. Wrapping her mother's quilt around herself, she opened it and found the
page she had last read. With trepidation, she turned the page.

May 27

I wonder if there can be an inverse response to a catharsis. A break-
down instead of a breakthrough? Cynthia was a little worried about
me, I know, after the session today when I couldn't talk. I sat in my
usual chair and watched her—role reversal, the patient observing
the clinician—while she read the last entry in my journal. In our
previous sessions we've just talked. I used the journal as a way for me

to get the words out so that, in her safe little office, I can say what I have no other place to say.

But I couldn't say anything today. Yet, it has become imperative to tell my story. This journal has become my voice, and I find that it's helping. I think I expected her to be appalled by the end. Maybe recommend institutionalization for inpatient therapy. I watched the emotion rippling across her eyelids as she read. She isn't as objective as she lets on. Tree of heaven, that woman must hear it all.

Yet, her response was completely unexpected. She simply closed my journal softly, and held it in her lap, regarding me silently. I knew what she was doing—waiting for me to express how I was feeling. Screaming, crying, collapsing on the floor. But I couldn't let myself go like that. I knew if I allowed myself to feel what my brain had hidden in a deep recess, I wouldn't be able to function. I wouldn't have the capacity to care for my family. I would bury myself and my pain under the blankets behind a locked bedroom door.

I could see the clock behind me reflected in the window. There were only seven minutes left in the session. I could hold it together that long.

"I think this journaling is really working for you," she said five minutes later. "But I wonder why you stopped where you did. From these last sessions and your journaling, we've identified three traumas in your recent life, all within one week. Your husband's possible infidelity, your sister and brother-in-law's murder, and witnessing a violent man attack a woman and threaten you in a foreign land.

"But clearly there is more to this incident that you're not yet ready to talk about. And yet you're still here a year after all of that happened. I wonder why it took a year for you to seek out help. It may be that the anniversary of these occurrences brought you here. It may be that your hormones are still off-balance from giving birth.

Or perhaps there's some other trigger that is bringing on the symptoms. Perhaps a combination. You've done some very difficult work here these past few weeks, but we have more to do. I'd encourage you to find time in the next week to be refreshed. Take a walk in that forest that gives you solace, rock with that new baby, whatever gives you peace. And when you're ready, continue the story. I know it's difficult, but trust the process. I'm here for you and I won't let you drown."

"Trust the process," she says. How can I ever trust anything anymore? That should give us something to talk about next week.

Chapter 21

"Trust the wings." The disembodied voice spoke through my stupor. My clammy skin clung to a cold surface. My head ached and a metallic taste filled my mouth and nostrils. It was too much of an effort to think.

I lifted one sticky eyelid and found myself eye-to-compound-eye with a large fly just inches from my face on the floor. His multi-faceted eyes stared at me. He seemed somehow disappointed that I was eyeing him back, still alive despite the blood drying on the tiles beside me, any element of surprise lost. I tried the other eye. The lashes stuck to my cheek till I rolled my head further to the side. Still the insect observed, unperturbed.

His presence and form fascinated me. Filament legs balanced the hairy body just off the ground. Iridescence faintly colored his wings like the surface of a soap bubble.

I wondered how those filmy membranes could manage to lift its bulky body off the ground. No wonder it was on the floor, unmoving. My body, too, was supine, pressed down into the damp tiles. Impossibly heavy.

"Trust the wings" came again in a whisper.

151

My lids drooped closed and terra cotta filled my vision. Warm water, like that in an earthenware bowl sitting in the sun, seeped from my eyes. I sank further into the cool tiles, smelling the damp clay, soothing my scraped arms and the sharp pain in my collarbone on the uneven surface.

"Trust the wings." The voice was gently persuasive.

A buzz pierced the air. I opened my eyes to find that the fly had disappeared. I was alone on the floor, in an unfamiliar room. I sensed the change in the temperature and knew it was afternoon. Alone was good. The man was gone, taking with him his property and the payment that the loutish man required for Auralei's safety—the violation of my body.

But I realized that I had to move. Because I was alone. Auralei was gone. Yet, the fly's delicate wings had miraculously lifted his hairy body aloft. I had to trust my wings. I had to move. My flimsy limbs pressed against the tiles and I rose, naked and shaking, and banked toward the light pouring through the open door.

I found my niece in the courtyard, silently pushing bougainvillea blooms under the water in the cement pila with an accusatory finger. Miraculously, she had been left behind and I gathered her up into my trembling arms.

She didn't speak or cry for the next two days, until Cal met us at O'Hare. He thrust a plush toucan hopefully toward her limp arms. She spoke only to the toucan for nine months, until she had a new plaything.

Avy turned the page. Edges of torn paper fell from the binding, like fragments of birch bark. Like the remnants of her mother's life—of *her* life. The rest of the pages, like her mind, were blank.

Who tore out these pages? she wondered. Was it her mother—or did her father read what she wrote here and want to destroy it? The "plaything"—it must have meant *her*.

She absently gathered the fragile fallen pieces of her mother's life into a tiny pile beside her. They taunted her with what she had just learned and with the missing pieces she would never know. A voice she barely recognized as her own whispered:

"My father didn't want to be a father."

"Yet he was so much more than the man I thought he was."

"An aunt and uncle, that I never knew existed, were murdered in Honduras."

"My mother saved her niece—my cousin—my sister. By being raped."

And then it slapped her in the face—"A rapist might actually be my 'father.'"

Avy reached Kirk Park just as the sun melted into Lake Michigan. She left the car outside the locked gate and walked in over the thin crust of ice that covered the snow. She found small shelter from the wind beside a trash barrel and huddled on an exposed driftwood log. For warmth, she buried her hands in the pockets of her jacket and felt her gloves. Not much protection, but they'd help, she figured, and drew them over her hands. She fumbled with numb fingers through threadbare gloves, unzipped the collar of her jacket and pulled the hood out of its pocket and over her head. The northerly wind pressed it against her cheek. The faint scent of Scotch pine carried on the air from the sand dune behind her.

The lake was oddly quiet, except for an occasional snap. The shoreline ice had thawed, then quick-frozen during the early

December deep freeze. But now the winter's thick ice floes from farther north in the lake drifted toward the frozen shoreline. As her eyes adjusted to the night, she sensed silent movement sweeping south along the shore. She stood, hunched against the wind, and moved gingerly toward the lake, navigating via scattered sand oases in the snow. Ice still gripped the shoreline, but a dozen feet out a black waterway flowed, glistening in the pale moonlight. A mountain of ice squatted on the sandbar beyond like the beaten hull of a shipwreck. Chunks glided in slow procession in the current between, like flotsam snaking between the sandbar and the near shore.

Avy ambled southward along the shore, emptying her mind of all but the scene before her. A break in the sandbar formed an eddy where the ice floes were drawn into a torpid dance, She found herself hypnotized.

Was it the capriciousness of life, she wondered, that had drawn her into its eddying grip, spinning her around and tossing her out into a channel she hadn't intended? Was she now being propelled relentlessly in a stupor down a sluggish current in the wrong direction? Or had she been flung into the vast inscrutable expanse, lost and drifting perilously, in danger of colliding with a sandbar? Was she eddying in between?

Chapter 22

She reentered the city before dawn and pulled into the gravel lot of an all-night neighborhood diner, Jack's Joint. Through the filmy glass, she watched a heavyset man, bundled in a Carhartt utility jacket and Yukon cap with earflaps, gulping down a pile of scrambled eggs. A side of greasy sausages waited. In her benumbed state, it looked like comfort food and she stepped out of the car. That and the unlimited coffee the sign offered might begin to thaw her body, even if her heart remained cold and her brain was slush. It would at least give her nourishment to face another day that lacked a workday routine to occupy her mind and give her direction.

She slid into a booth near the kitchen and ordered coffee. The lone waitress brought a mug and a pot of steaming brew and hovered. Avy recognized that if she wanted to stay, she needed to order breakfast. She managed to stretch the scrambled eggs and pancakes out as long as she could, and asked for another pot of coffee. The sun rose as she poured the last of the cold brew into her mug. A new waitress arrived for the day shift and Avy ordered an English muffin and orange juice as the night shift girl headed out into the cold.

Body warmed, and propelled by the coffee, Avy used the restroom and left the diner. Not yet ready to return to the house, she found herself wandering on foot through an unfamiliar part of the city as people with purpose headed into their day.

Chimes rang nearby, a familiar tune. Avy drifted in their direction. Ahead, a stooped, gray-haired woman shuffled, wrestling a grocery cart filled with bulging black garbage bags and missing a rear wheel. A caramel-colored cat perched atop a duffle bag crammed in the child-seat, her eyes jouncing wide with each jolt of the uneven pavement. Avy overtook them as the woman settled herself on a wooden bench opposite a church. Trinity Episcopal, the engraved limestone read.

Avy sat too. She was so tired. Her car, she knew, was still parked at the diner, but she had lost track of where the diner was. She would stumble back onto it eventually. There was no reason to look for it now. No reason to get in and drive. No reason to act and every reason to postpone action.

The woman beside her was dressed in layers that carried the acrid odor of cat pee. A gray sweatshirt peeked through the eyelet holes in an oversized cardigan sweater colored a faded turquoise. From the stretched-out neck of the sweatshirt, a red turtleneck bunched. Leopard leggings hugged her calves, disappearing under cut-off Army fatigues. Her bare ankles were swollen and pitted with scabs above pink ballet slippers. Avy saw all this while she pointedly ignored the woman's open stare.

Across the street, a few cars funneled into the church parking lot. A striking woman, dressed in black palazzo pants and a fiery caftan that set off the cinnamon hue of her skin, strode up the wide stone steps and pulled open the heavy door. A figure shadowed in the entry wrapped its gray-suited arm around her as the door swung closed behind them. Faint organ music hung in the air like a memory.

She wondered what it would be like to be welcomed by that arm. To rest in that place.

"Are you a giving person?" The woman sitting beside her broke into her reverie.

"I'm a nurse," Avy said curtly, staring at the wooden door. That should say it all, she felt.

"I go in there sometimes," the woman remarked. "I know *all* the churches 'round here. As churches go, this one's a giving church."

"What do you mean? They give you money?" Avy asked.

"Hah! They're not *that* giving." The woman sniggered. "But they do give me food sometimes, and I got this sweater there. When my teeth were paining me like a hot poker, they got 'em pulled for me. They let me stay in the shelter with Precious here. Most places, they don't allow animals."

They watched then, in silence, as a few more parishioners entered the church, but the parking lot had plenty of room left over. Not unusual for a Saturday morning. In fact, what are these people doing there on a Saturday anyway? she wondered. Choir practice? That could explain the organ music.

"You see that black lady go in a bit ago? She's some kind of psychic or something. I seen 'er a couple times. For a black lady, she's pretty smart. She knows how to talk to doctors and stuff. She got me some pills but I run out. I have to talk to her again if I want some more but I don't like to take charity from no black lady. At the clinic downtown, they say I got afro-sclerosis. She's the only negro I ever had any truck with so I must've caught it from her." Avy turned her head just enough to cast a side-glance at her companion. Her face, in profile, stared noncommittally at the limestone blocks of the church.

"So now I just ignore the voices. She told me I could. It's okay, she said. Most people, they ignore me, so it's fair I get to ignore somebody too."

"Maybe I should talk to her," Avy mumbled. "I'm having a real hard time ignoring certain voices lately."

"Here," the woman said, digging in a canvas flight bag, "I got 'er card here. I don't need it anymore. You want it?"

Avy absently tucked the card in her pocket, felt some coins, and pulled them out to give the woman.

"God bless you, and Josie thanks you. I knew you were a giving person." She held Avy's hand a little longer than was necessary as thanks for pocket change. Avy stood and turned away. "And it's okay to ignore the voices," the woman called out as Avy retraced her steps.

Chapter 23

Thanksgiving had passed unnoticed by her father. Avy didn't have the energy to stage a celebratory meal for just the two of them, anyway. Besides, she wasn't feeling particularly thankful. Maybe when she got to Albany she'd have something to appreciate. And people to celebrate with.

Instead, she'd spent the past few days looking into options for her father's care and her peace of mind in order to leave him. Dr. Nanninga had given him both a physical and mental exam, taken blood, reordered all his medications, and confirmed that he had some type of dementia. "It doesn't present as typical Alzheimer's, but certainly something has deteriorated in his brain function." He made a referral for a neuro consult and further tests. Before leaving the office, she had the letter she needed and a packet of information on local elder care services. There were options, but it would be a battle to get him to agree to any of them.

First, there was institutionalization. Extended care seemed like a great option. Until she saw the price tag. She still hadn't found any financial records in the house, but it had to be out of his reach to afford the kind of services they offered. Medicare didn't begin to cover what he would need—medication management, housekeeping, room and board, personal care. And then, as his memory got worse, specialized dementia care. Besides, he'd never agree to it.

So, she considered, extra care in the home. A nurse to set up medications once a week in a med box—something new for him to remember. Housekeeping—someone invading his space and touching his belongings. Grocery shopping—maybe that would be acceptable if he'd let them put it all away where it belonged; but would he eat properly even if it was there? Personal care—out of the question. And that still wouldn't guarantee he wouldn't wander off or get into the kind of trouble she'd faced on her arrival at his home.

There was adult daycare, she thought. Another new place. Driving. It would give him socialization, but he'd have to get himself there. Maybe the place had a van, but would he accept a ride? He'd get one meal there, but what about the rest of his meals? And it wouldn't help with his erratic medication use. Plus he could wander off there, too, just as easily. And then he'd be lost in unfamiliar surroundings.

Live-in help would be ideal, but he'd never agree to having someone in his home—just look at how he'd resented *her* presence, she thought. And who else would put up with him? Only a saint. And then—a stroke of genius—a wife! That's a laugh!

Still, something had to be done. She had less than a week left to make his house as safe as possible for him to continue living alone. It was the only way she could leave without carrying guilt along with her into her resurrected life.

What was it in her that had to take responsibility, she wondered, when neither Jared nor Auralei felt any remorse for abandoning him? But then, she'd been able to erase him for ten years, too. "Chicory!"

Avy bought a weekly med box, recommended by the Rite Aid pharmacist when she picked up her father's newly ordered prescriptions. While there, she ordered a medical bracelet, although she doubted he would consent to wear it.

The Staples store proved to be the mother lode of inspiration. She asked the bored teen, picking off her glitter nail polish at the service desk, to copy and retouch some old family photos. While she waited for the photos, she wandered the aisles. Among the plethora of office merchandise, her eyes lit on a label maker. She grabbed it and four colors of label tape, a multipack of sticky notes, a whiteboard with markers, a new Tigers Baseball calendar for the year 2000. She had to return to the entrance for a basket in order to manage it all, plus a talking alarm clock with several different reminder modes. It was styled as a 1950s Motorola upright radio. She figured he'd love it.

Back home, Avy filled the med box, hoping it would help. She called a local home care agency to inquire about services and set up an interview for later that week. It was worth a try.

Her father found the clock and its reminders offensive at first, but he did like its incongruously retro style. Predictably, he ignored his medication box sitting conspicuously on the kitchen table. When the clock sounded a reminder, he became deaf. Avy was convinced he did it just to annoy her, and she would stare at him until he felt it, looked up, and calmly opened the lid for the pills. Sometimes he would take pills out of the wrong slot while she watched, and again she thought he was baiting her. But by the end of the week, he had agreed that the "pretty nurse" who had interviewed him could come once a week to fill it up again.

Avy had engaged the nurse from Alliance Homecare. The agency was highly recommended by Dr. Nanninga and also by the pharmacist at Rite Aid, and that service was covered by Medicare. He also agreed that a household helper could come once a week, even though he would have to pay for it, to clean the house and do the laundry. "That's woman's work anyway, and it would give me more time to do my research," he declared, forgetting that was how Avy had couched the proposal.

By the end of the week, Avy's labels colored every cabinet, refrigerator shelf, closet, and drawer. She posted pictures of the family with their names and phone numbers on the refrigerator door. She returned the whiteboard and markers to Staples, but the calendar hung proudly on the wall.

She had done what she could, and Jared would be home for Christmas break to see if her plan was successful. Now she could focus on packing for her departure.

She needed a few additional clothing items to flesh out an executive wardrobe. Shopping for clothes and shoes was anathema to her—she puzzled how she and Auralei could be so different; then remembered that, of course, they weren't really sisters! Yet she was pleased with her new, stylishly understated black suit with an open-front jacket. So she accessorized with a handful of bright blouses and camisoles and new black leather pumps with a more up-to-date heel. Then, on a haughty pale mannequin, posed with her hands resting on forward-thrust hips, she saw the dress. Cerulean blue silk, ruched—she thought that was the word for it—V-neck bodice, with a mid-calf A-line skirt that floated in the breeze of passing shoppers. It called for splurging on some silky lingerie, too.

She fumbled in her bag for her wallet, and her hand found the citrine crystal Auralei had given her. Yes, her professional life was getting back on track. She could practically feel her chakras opening.

Chapter 24

Avy felt a sense of déjà vu as she stared at her image in the reflective surface of the elevator. Her amber eyes glinted like two
tiger's-eye gemstones, translucent and focused, highlighted with
mascara and dusky eye shadow. Her matte black eyeglass frames
enhanced her updated look and gave her an air of authority. At her
throat, an opal pendant glistened on its silver choker, like a gibbous
moon above the teal blouse. Matching opal ear studs shone like
twin stars against her black hair. She had augmented her usual clear
gloss with a new shade of lipstick—Triumphant Taupe. The elevator doors slid open and she strode out in her new suit and heels.

She hesitated to even think of the phrase she had used only
a month ago at Denver's Saint Stephen's—that this was the day
all her hard work would pay off. But now it *had* paid off. Her
ten-year goal, chief nursing officer—never mind that it was in a
new locale—was realized. She was "onboarding." And it was only
December 13.

She entered the executive suite and stopped at the secretary's
desk to introduce herself. The secretary—Sharon, according to the
nameplate on the desk—excused herself to inform the HR manager

of her early arrival. Avy glanced in her direction as Sharon passed through the office suite, but her eyes were arrested by a door with a brass plate—Aviana Lehrer, RN, MSN, Chief Nursing Officer. She could see through the frosted glass that it already held a desk with a smoky glass top resting upon arcing matte-black supports, a black Aeron chair, a small matching conference table and chairs, a black file cabinet, and empty glass bookshelves. A vase of red roses gave the room a burst of color.

Silently, she vowed that she would be celebrating the turn of the century in that office.

She roused herself as a slim man, in a gray suit that matched his hair, stepped from his office.

"Ms. Lehrer, welcome." His eyes seemed to rest on the choker settled in the suprasternal notch of her throat, before jerking back up to her eyes. "I'm Ted Carson, HR manager. So happy to have you join us. Let's get this ball rolling, shall we?"

She gripped his outstretched hand and gave a sharp nod of her head.

"Let's. I couldn't wish for anything more."

She followed him back into his office, where a thick binder awaited her on his desk. Her new life was about to begin.

Chapter 25

Several Christmas cards from her new colleagues took the place of family photos on Avy's desk—impersonal, gold-embossed season's greetings. Notably, there were none from her life before December 13, not even from her brother, but then almost no one knew where she was except her father—if he remembered—the home care agency, Jared, Auralei, Andrew. That was it. When she left Denver she really had no friends there to wonder about her and she, in turn, never thought of her former colleagues. She'd left a message with Auralei, giving her contact information, but so far had received no response. She thought maybe she should tell her that she'd upgraded her wardrobe or that the crystal helped her get this new job. . . .

Having just begun her new position, she wouldn't be getting time off except for Christmas Day, but she would have liked to have *some* kind of holiday celebration—she'd even settle for a celebratory dinner with her snooty sister. The hospital Christmas party was understated—a buffet that ran from 11:00 till 4:00. By the time she broke away to go to the party, the remaining ham and asparagus roll-ups looked pitiful, the asparagus limp and the ham slices curling at the edges. She squirreled away a couple of mint-chocolate brownies, drank some undoctored eggnog, and returned to her office.

Two new envelopes waited on her desk. One, marked with the logo for Alliance Homecare, was in an overnight envelope. Probably the first bill, she thought. The other was in Jared's handwriting. She opened his first, a card that bore a winter photograph of the Rockefeller Chapel on the Chicago campus. Inside was the greeting, "Merry Christmas from the Windy City!" Then a scribbled note, "I got an invitation to Snowbird Ski Resort over the holidays, so I'm headed off to Utah! Hope you're settling in to the new position in old New York! Stay warm and drink some grog for me! Cheers! Jared."

"Bittercress!" She threw the card on the desk, where a corner slid under the other envelope from the home care company. "He skipped out on Christmas with Dad!" She'd counted on Jared and didn't have the holiday covered with the Alliance helpers. She hoped they could still schedule it. She grabbed the oblong envelope and tore it open. On Alliance letterhead was a brief statement:

"We are unable to continue to fill your request for nursing or household help as the patient has threatened our staff on numerous occasions, made an accusation of theft, and inappropriately touched one of our nurses. The police have investigated and concluded that there is no evidence that the theft occurred, but we cannot be put in this position again. Attached you will find our bill for the three weeks that we were involved."

"Oh, toadflax! Mugwort! Sweet *Lythrum salicaria!*" Footsteps outside her office paused briefly, then padded on.

Escalating to the scientific names of invasive species to express her anger was a bad sign. She willed Jared to hit a tree on a black diamond run and break both legs. *"Cirsium vulgare!"* she rasped out as quietly as she could. It sounded like a witch's curse.

Finally, Avy picked up the phone, dialed Dale Monfort's office, and heard, "The office is closed for the holiday. Please leave a message at the tone and we will return your call when we reopen on Thursday, January 2."

"Mr. Monfort, this is Aviana Lehrer. I'm calling from New York, where I've just started that new position I mentioned. Alliance Homecare has quit caring for Dad, and Jared decided to go skiing instead of going home to spend time with him. I'm at a loss what to do from here without the proper authority. Please call me as soon as possible."

She left the message with her cell phone number in hopes that he might still return her call, but she had immediate responsibilities to focus on. She grabbed a stack of folders and the agenda for her first meeting with the unit managers at 3:30, stood from her ergonomic chair, and loosened the skirt that had attached itself to her stockings like a second skin. She closed her eyes for a moment and took a deep breath. And another. She forced her shoulders to unlock, slapped a smile on her face, then walked briskly from her office.

Chapter 26

"Avy. It's Andrew again. I seem to be making a habit of calling you at odd hours. Maybe I should have waited, but I wanted to catch you before you started work, assuming that as a newbie you didn't get the holiday off."

Avy rubbed the sleep from her eyes and reached for her glasses.

"Andrew. Hi. Why do I know that this isn't a call with good news?" She wrangled her glasses on with one hand and checked the time: 5:26 a.m. She swung her legs out from under her new down comforter and sat on the side of the bed.

"Well, your instincts are on target. We got a call from your father's neighbor, Mrs. Graham, early this morning. It's not the first time. In the past, she's called to complain about the dog running around loose and fouling her garden, but this time she woke up to what she surmised was a smoke alarm. She called us because it was still going after fifteen minutes and her dog was howling under her bed and keeping her awake."

"She waited fifteen minutes?" Avy rubbed her forehead with her free hand. "Why didn't she alert the fire department right away instead of finally calling the police?"

"Exactly what I asked her." He suppressed a laugh. "She claimed she opened her window when the alarm didn't stop and she didn't see or smell smoke, so she knew it wasn't a fire."

"And was it?"

"No. Fortunately, it turned out she was right, but I called the fire department to check on it, then met them there. No smoke. No fire. No answer to knocking at the door, but it wasn't locked, so we called out and went in. I don't know how he could have slept through that din, but he did. I went upstairs to make sure he was there and that he was okay. He was snoring away under a load of blankets. I suspect he may have been drinking again. Alex crept out from under the bed, whining. I believe he remembered me."

"So what caused it?"

"You're not going to like it."

"Of course I'm not going to like it, Andrew! Just tell me and get it over with!"

"When the firemen took the smoke alarm down to reset it, the inside was caked with grease and cobwebs—and dead bugs. That, plus its age, set it off."

"Please tell me it wasn't cockroaches!"

"I didn't ask for specifics, but I don't think so."

Avy sighed. "This just gets better and better. I found out last week that the home care agency I hired quit. He was obnoxious and threatening to their staff. I plan to try to hire another, but without me there to introduce them and make sure he lets them in . . . I don't know what else to do." She plowed her fingers through her hair in frustration, gripping a clump and pulling till her eyes teared. "Jared was supposed to be there over his college break, but he went skiing instead."

"Well, I wrote up my visit officially as a police wellness check. Other than the mess and the smoke alarm, I didn't see anything that would cause me to be overly worried. He's clearly eating, because there was plenty of evidence in the sink and on the table. And the food in his fridge was okay. Oh—and there was no sign of dog poop or pee, so he seems to be getting Alex out to do his duty regularly—although the dog was desperate to get out this morning—which means he must be giving him food and water."

"Thank God for that. I'm worried about his meds, though, if he's taking them the way he should. The nurse was supposed to be setting them up each week and monitoring that."

"I don't know about his meds, but if you can tell me what he's supposed to be taking I can do another wellness check and see."

"Yes, please! That would really help. I expect the med box on the kitchen table may be empty, but who knows. The pill bottles were in the cupboard beside the fridge, but again, I have no idea where they might be now."

"You know what, Avy?" His voice had a lighter note. "I have an idea. Mom's a retired nurse. Maybe she'd be willing to look in on him once or twice a week." Andrew's voice turned hesitant. "He might remember her from when we were in high school."

"I doubt that he'd remember, but I'd be grateful if she's willing to try. I can fax you a list of his meds if she could check that out—there should be a list there, too, that the nurse was to use. And he was supposed to have housekeeping help through the agency, but I suppose that fell through, too. Anything you can think of would be a blessing, Andrew. I would really appreciate it. And of course I'll pay her whatever seems fair."

"Right. I can't promise anything, but I'll see what I can do. But, hey! How's the new job going? How's Albany?"

"I've just been getting organized at work, but I love the hospital and the people here are great. I think it was a blessing in disguise that I missed out on the promotion in Denver."

"You didn't tell me that you were up for a promotion there. I'm sorry you didn't get it, but it sounds like you've landed on your feet."

"I have, Andrew!" Her voice rang. "I had a ten-year plan to achieve a nurse administrator position by the year 2000, and I've done it! I feel like a phoenix rising from the ashes of that disaster." She laughed in mild embarrassment at the stretched idiom, but found herself practically dancing across the hardwood floor of her sparsely furnished apartment.

"That's great, Avy. You deserve whatever good is coming to you! And let me be the first to wish you a Happy New Year—unless you were out partying last night, kissing the first guy in sight at midnight."

"Ha! You know me so well. Happy New Year to you, too, Andrew."

Over the phone, his strong baritone rang out. "Should old acquaintance be forgot . . ."

"And never brought to mind," she joined in with gusto, squeaking a bit as she reached the limit of her alto voice. They finished together: "Should old acquaintance be forgot, and days of auld lang syne."

"I don't have a clue what auld lang syne means." She laughed. "Did you and I have days of auld lang syne?"

"Something like old time's sake, I think. Don't forget old friends and old times as you look forward to the new."

"Appropriate, old friend."

"I'm glad we caught up again, even though it's been a difficult time for you."

"I am, too. Thanks, Andrew. For old times and for what you're willing to do for me now. I won't forget again."

"I'll be in touch, Avy, to let you know if Mom can help. But keep moving forward into this new time and place for you. I wish you all the best."

She waited till her phone indicated he'd hung up. She closed it and held it to her chest, a wistful smile spreading upward to her eyes. In her rush to escape from her father's house years ago, she'd put old friends and good times out of her mind as if folding up outworn clothes in a trunk, never to be opened. Andrew had been a faithful friend then. Despite her rudeness to him recently, his loyalty to their friendship was proving itself again. He was a sweetheart.

She resumed her seat on the bed and wrapped herself in her mother's quilt, taken from her father's house. She had heard that odors could evoke memories and emotions and had found it to be true. She had often breathed deeply into the quilt, to inhale the familiar fecund fragrance, like that of a garden, dewy, earthy, and sweet. It evoked both a comfort and a melancholy for the mother she had lost. Now she noted another scent that rose from it. She had smelled it before, but now it struck her as different, reminiscent not just of her mother, but of something else as well, that she'd always neglected to consider—the somewhat stale, buttered-toast smell of popcorn—which she had enjoyed years ago, cuddled under the quilt in front of the TV, with Andrew. She hugged the quilt up to her cheeks to hold back unexpected tears.

Chapter 27

On an unusually warm January day, a crisp thirty-six degrees, but windless and sunny, a bluebird sky urged her upward into the Catskills toward Windham High Peak. She sloshed through a few muddy spots along the trail that appeared to be more of a creek bed, given the occasional rivulets of pristine water flowing across the rocky path. Her mother's hiking boots gripped the uneven ground and, along with a maple-branch hiking pole, kept her upright. The knapsack on her back held a thermos of coffee, a Swiss Army knife, and a trail map she had printed off at work. She had thought to tuck in two extra pairs of socks, knowing they might be needed in the wet terrain, but wore the nubby wool ones she had kept for so many years. Her mother's binoculars hung from her neck.

Avy's mother seemed to walk beside her as she made her way steadily upward. "Mom, you would love this place," she shared aloud, sitting to rest on a boulder near the lean-to, identified by a triangle on her map. "It's just magical here, carpeted in pockets of snow and maple leaves that still hint at their fall colors. I've been walking through a silent winter forest, exposed roots spreading out

over the ground, tripping over themselves—and occasionally tripping me! I can almost sense the mycelium threads spreading in
their underground network, giving the trees nourishment to last
the winter." She breathed deeply. "The smells, Mom: earth, leaf
decay, the crisp citrusy smell of the spruce trees." She wished her
mother was seated beside her. "I miss you so much. Thank you for
all that you taught me so I could appreciate this world like you did."

She finished her coffee and dropped the thermos back in the
knapsack, but she was in no hurry to move on. The entrancing view
and the mystical sense of her mother's presence kept her in place,
basking in the sun. She was unwilling to break the spell.

She raised the binoculars to her eyes and trained the focus on
an ancient birch tree with an unusual outgrowth near its scraggy
top. A barred owlet, embraced by the striated feathers of its mother's breast, peered back at her. Her breath caught in her throat.
She experienced a fleeting sensation of a soft touch on her cheek.
Warmth flowed from it into her body, spreading through her arteries to her heart. Her hand flew to her chest and an amazed cry
escaped from her throat. She jumped up, reenergized, and hoisted
the knapsack onto her back. In silence again, she hiked on, reflecting that in a place like this, God might actually exist.

Chapter 28

While waiting for Andrew's weekly Wednesday report, Avy stood gazing out her fifth-floor office window. She blocked out this hour in her schedule in order to be apprised of how Andrew and his mother had found her father that week. Thanks to her old friend, she could concentrate fully on her challenging work, but she looked forward to this weekly break in her day, relishing the glorious view from her window and the sense of relief that Andrew's call always brought. To the west, Windham High Peak shone, frosted in fresh powder from last night's snowfall. It wasn't the view of Mount Evans that she'd enjoyed months ago in Denver, but it had become her favorite sight this winter.

As she relived that hike six weeks ago and observed her reflection in the window's glass, a smile softened her face. She wondered how the owlet and its mother were faring. Her reverie was interrupted by the ring of her cell phone on the desk behind her.

"Hey, Andrew! Punctual as usual. How's it going back in Berndtbridge?"

"Hey, Avy. Don't worry; your Dad's fine. Mom's had him eating out of her hand, but—"

"That's wonderful, Andrew. Please let her know how grateful I am."

"Of course. I'll pass that on, but there *is* a problem." She held her breath, waiting for Andrew to continue. "I found Mom unconscious in her bedroom when I stopped by after work this morning. I'm with her at the ER right now. She's had some sort of an incident, they're saying. They think she may have had a stroke—or a seizure?"

"Oh—that's terrible!" she cried. "What are her symptoms? Did they give her tPA? Who's the doc?"

"Avy, slow down. You know I have no idea what you're talking about. She's had a couple of doctors in to evaluate her, and she's got an IV going in her arm. Is that the PTA you're talking about?"

"tPA. Look at the bag of fluid that's running and tell me what it says."

"Um. A nurse just came in. Let me just ask her."

Avy heard Andrew's muffled voice speaking to the nurse; then, "Yes, she says it's a medicine to break up a blood clot—sounds like 'All-the-place'?—something like that. She's nodding at me—and trying not to laugh."

"Alteplase. That's it. Good. So, is your Mom awake? Can she talk? Move her fingers and toes? Smile?"

"She's awake now, but her words aren't making sense. She seems angry—or maybe frustrated? I don't know. I watched one of the doctors try to get her to follow his finger with his eyes. I don't know how successful that was, but I did see her push against his hands with her feet when he asked her to. What does it all mean, Avy? I'm lost here."

Avy drew a breath to settle her thoughts, and calm Andrew down, too. He was asking for her opinion as a friend and a professional even though a nurse was there in the room with him. She needed to answer like the professional she was.

"Everything you're telling me does sound a lot like a stroke, although I don't want to diagnose from across the country. Alteplase is the drug given to break up a clot, which is what causes a stroke. Giving it quickly after the symptoms start reduces the possibility of long-term effects like slurred speech and weakness. The symptoms you describe are common for a stroke, too. They may linger, but with the Alteplase and therapy, she may completely recover."

"That's good to hear."

"She's in good hands, Andrew. Yours and the hospital staff. Berndtbridge Memorial, for a small local hospital, has a good reputation, and they'll make sure she gets what she needs, both in the hospital and for aftercare when she leaves. If she's able to go home right from the hospital she should qualify for home care, but they may have to send her to a rehab facility first."

She heard Andrew's breath draw in and blow out over the phone. She hoped she wasn't increasing his fears, on the one hand, or giving him false confidence, on the other.

"Thanks, Avy. It's reassuring to hear that, but I'm still worried."

"I won't tell you not to worry, Andrew. That's not reasonable. But I'll support you in any way I can from here. Call me whenever."

"Yeah, okay. Thanks, again."

She hesitated, but had to ask. "Will you still be able to check on my Dad?"

"Of course. I think Mom got him set up for the week with pills and food just yesterday. I'll let you know if there are any problems."

"You're the best, Andrew. When things calm down there at the hospital, give your mom my best wishes for a quick recovery. I'll be thinking of you both and sending good vibes."

"Thanks, Avy. Hang on a sec." His voice became muffled, then returned. "They're taking her now for an MRI. Is that good?"

"Yes. That's an important test to confirm the stroke and direct further treatment. I'll let you go now, so you can keep track of everything there, okay?"

"Yeah, Thanks again. Talk later."

As she hung up she made a mental note to send flowers. Mrs. Chase was such a dear soul. The widow had enfolded Avy into her life when she and Andrew had been a thing in their senior year. It hadn't in any way made up for her own mom, but still. It was painful to think of her so disabled and afraid.

Avy's nose tickled with the memory of the s'more's brownie aroma that hung in the air back then. She decided that she needed chocolate right away and strode through her office door toward the cafeteria. The packaged brownies in the machine, while nothing like Mrs. Chase's, would have to do. Maybe two packages.

Chapter 29

It wasn't a stroke. The MRI instead had shown a murky tumor in the right temporal area. A meningioma. A brain tumor masquerading as a stroke. Avy wished she could airlift Lydia to Saint Catherine's for treatment, but Berndtbridge's team had already put a plan in motion.

Andrew's hastily granted week's leave did not include his unauthorized police escort for the ambulance transferring his mother to the University of Michigan cancer center in Ann Arbor. Lydia's surgery began three hours after her arrival. Andrew updated Avy every hour while he paced between the cafeteria and the waiting room.

Avy decided to adjust her plan: thanks to Valentine's Day and Presidents' Day hugging the shoulders of the weekend, Avy had managed a four-day break to check on her father. She already had a suitcase packed and stashed in her trunk. She left the hospital that evening at 5:30 and drove into the night. Heading west, she navigated south of Lake Erie instead of through Canada. It was a longer route, but Buffalo had been hit with a snowstorm and roads were closed at the border until the plows could clear it. She'd

learned to respect the Midwest's winter storms since her trip across
the border in November.

⸺⬦⬦⬦⸺

At the door to Lydia's hospital room, Avy stopped, her eyes adjusting to the dim light. Andrew slept in a chair by his mother's
bedside, head crooked awkwardly toward his shoulder. His face,
relaxed in sleep, had dropped the mask of authority he wore in his
profession. She saw him again as a vulnerable, insecure high school
student, an eager-to-please youth who, she knew, had adored her.
She felt herself drawn to touch his shoulder, but resisted. Instead,
she took a seat on the bed beside Lydia.

The woman's head was swathed with gauze, her mouth slack in
sleep. Tape held oxygen tubing to her cheek and Avy could hear the
soft whoosh as the air entered Lydia's nostrils. A blood pressure cuff
inflated with a loud hum and she waited for the figures to appear
on the monitor—126 over 72. Her pulse beat steadily at 66 and the
oxygen was at 94. All within normal limits. The IV bag dripped
fluids and antibiotic steadily into her antecubital vein. With fingers
as gentle as a breath, Avy traced the tendons of the woman's hand
from fingers to wrist, content to share this quiet space of recovery.

"Eebee." The voice was soft as a whisper. Avy inclined over her
as Lydia's eyes searched her face with puzzlement.

"Yes, it's Avy. Andrew told me what happened. I'm so sorry
you're going through this." She brought the woman's hand to her
lips and kissed it. "Andrew's sleeping right here."

"Not anymore," he said. He stood stiffly and steadied himself
with a hand on the bed rail. "Thanks for coming," he said. Avy
smiled up at him, released Lydia's hand, and slid off the bed to give
him space to approach.

"Mom, it's great to see you awake. You remember Avy? She's been on the phone with me while you've been going through this, but she wanted to be here to see how you were."

Lydia looked from Andrew to Avy and moved her bandaged head in a small nod. Then she turned back to Andrew with a creased brow. Andrew sat on the bed where Avy had just been and she moved to sit across from him.

"Your tumor was benign, Mom, and the surgeon believes they were able to get the entire mass out, but plan to follow up with routine MRI's just in case. That's the standard treatment." He glanced at Avy for confirmation. "You'll be able to go home in a few days. How does that sound?"

Lydia closed one eye and scrunched up her nose.

"What does *that* mean?" Andrew asked. She stuck out her tongue, then licked her dry lips. "Jus' dandy," she managed.

Avy laughed aloud. "You're going to have your hands full, Andrew." She winked at Lydia. "Has anyone talked to you about what you can expect she'll need when you go home?"

"I haven't thought that far ahead," he admitted, "but they did say she would have a physical therapist coming in today to assess her abilities and get her moving." Avy nodded and turned back to Lydia.

"Lydia, assuming you're able to go home in a few days, you'll probably need help." Lydia rolled her eyes as if to say, "Duh!" Avy grinned. "You should be able to have a nurse and a therapist visit you at home, but you'll probably need more help than that. I'm guessing they won't want you to be alone."

"I'm going to stay with Mom as long as she needs me. My boss is looking into FMLA, but it would be a real hardship on them for me to take more time off. It's such a small department. But she's looking into what we can work out. I do have to work on Sunday, though. If she goes home that day, is there any chance that you could be at the house? When do you have to return to New York?"

"I've got Monday off for the holiday, so I'll be driving back that day, but if she comes home on Sunday, I can get her settled." Avy wondered if it would be enough time, though. Would Lydia be strong enough to leave the hospital so soon? People recovered in different ways and times from brain surgery. One day at a time, she counseled herself. She reached into her bag for her wallet. "Here's the card for Alliance, the home care company that was with Dad. Even though they discharged him, I would still recommend them. It was Dad's behavior, not their lack of skill, that was the problem." Andrew took the card. "The hospital discharge planner will come in today or tomorrow, probably, to get the plan going. They should go with whatever agency you choose."

Avy spent a few more minutes with them, but she was anxious to finish the trip to Berndtbridge to check on her father. She dreaded what she might find.

Chapter 30

After banging on the door and ringing the bell to no avail, the frustration of standing, freezing in the snow on the stoop of her old home, took over. It was barely light, and she hadn't slept in hours. She muttered to herself, why now does he finally begin to lock the door? She shivered. But Alex, barking in a frenzy, scrabbled at the door from inside. She sensed that something was definitely off. There used to be a spare key hidden behind a 1x4 spanning the studs in the garage. She hoped it was still there as she trudged through the wet snow.

The garage side door opened partway into the dingy space, enough to poke her head through and find a banged-up, lidless metal trash can blocking her entrance. She shoved harder and squeezed inside. The door bounced shut behind her. The smell told her something had been left to rot in there.

She turned her back on the trash can. Her eyes adjusted to the darkness and picked out her father's Buick crammed between Jared's old Schwinn, the grass-encrusted Toro, a spare tire leaning against the wall, warped 2x4s that she knew had been in the same spot forever, two rickety wooden stepladders hanging on the far wall with an assortment of tools, and a potting bench with her mother's gardening paraphernalia, which hadn't been touched for ten years. A web-sprung lawn chair was smashed between the front bumper and the overhead door.

The 1x4 was still nailed in place on the wall as if holding the old structure together. The window above it was only a window in name, not function. It was so grimy that only a dusky light pushed through to highlight the intricate spiderwebs encasing it and the spot behind which she hoped the key still hung. Her nose wrinkled, scrunching her glasses up to her eyebrows. She searched for something to clear the webs and any spiders that crouched there, and her eyes lit on a rusty leaf rake splayed underneath the car. The tines squealed across the cement floor like fingernails on a chalkboard as she dragged it out from beneath the car. Her ears vibrated from the sound.

The rake worked like a charm, though, drawing the wispy threads by its tines, screeching across the glass like a hawk's cry. She had to climb over the lawnmower to angle the rake behind the board. She wasn't really afraid of spiders per se. Her mother had taught her well, but still, they were creepy and she didn't want one landing on her hand when she felt for the key.

She was just about to reach behind the crosspiece when the spider dropped on its filament to disappear into the darkness. She knocked the rake handle against the board, hoping any lingering critters got the message that it was time to leave and, for good measure, she cajoled them with a promise of a better life in the open air.

Finally, her fingers crept behind the board and, as if by memory, immediately found the nail with the key hanging from it. She blew off the dust and hiked her leg back over the lawnmower to head into the open air herself.

She slogged back to the house, sneezing out dust in triple gusts of breath and snot. She wiped her nose with her coat sleeve. At the front door, fitting the rusty key in the lock, she felt Alex's fren-zied battering of the door from inside. His body squirmed through the narrow slit as the door opened and he leapt from the stoop into the patch of pachysandra poking through the blanket of snow to relieve himself as she waited. Then, as she stepped across the threshold, he came barreling back inside and threw himself at her legs, nearly toppling her onto the wooden floor.

She caught her balance and reached down to receive his wel-coming slobbers. "Aw, are you my sweet boy? Happy Valentine's Day, buddy!" She began to scratch his chin, but he cocked his head at her, then spun and dashed upstairs. She scurried after him.

The bedclothes resembled her recent view of the Catskills—low mounds of gentle foothills—and she approached cautiously, call-ing out, "Dad? Dad? You in there somewhere?" She was rewarded with a grunt followed by hacking coughs emanating from under the blankets, and a shifting of the mounds. The face scowling up at her was flushed and moist, the hair a greasy mat, and the odor of sweat and urine overpowering.

"Oh, spurge," she murmured. "You're sick," she said aloud.

"Says who?"

She reached across the bed to remove some of the bedclothes. His hand whipped out from under the blankets, landing across her face. Reeling, she nearly tripped over the dog at her feet. The slap brought her back to her seventeen-year-old self, when she'd last felt that burning flesh and vowed to plan her escape.

"What are you doing here? Can't you just mind your own busi-ness and leave an old man alone?" he growled.

"No, I can't," she replied, as tears threatened to fall. The urge to slap him back, as she had once done, warred with her adult self-possession and her Pavlovian response to treat illness. "I need to check your temp and listen to your lungs."

"Not a chance!"

"You can't just lie here. Let's get you sitting up so I can check you out and change the bedding and your clothes."

"Get out of my way. I have to pee."

"Great, first things first. I'll go get the thermometer and start a bath so you can soak in the tub for a bit to clear your lungs."

"I have to pee!" he shouted, and convulsed with another fit of coughing. When the coughing settled into a wheezing sputter of shallow breaths, he glared at her. The scent of concentrated urine rose. He was soaked.

"Okay. Let's get you to the bathroom."

"I don't want you ogling me!"

"Don't worry. I've seen it all. But I promise not to look."

"I don't need your help anyway. I can pee myself."

Yes, she agreed silently, you've clearly peed yourself. "Alright. I'll just stand by in case you do need me."

"I won't."

"Okay."

He hoisted himself out of bed and waved her away. She stepped back, letting him walk alone, but with her body on alert to catch him should he begin to fall. He stumbled into the bathroom and slammed the door in her face.

"Okay."

Avy went into efficiency nursing mode. She stripped the bed down to the mattress, flew to the top of the stairs, tossed the whole bundle to the bottom, and returned to the bathroom door.

"You okay in there?"

"Go away!"

So she did. Back to the hallway linen closet, where she grabbed a sheet set for his double bed, and two blankets. There was no spare mattress pad, so she pulled out one more blanket to substitute.

The toilet flushed. She waited, and heard water running—and running. Then the tub stopper thunked into place.

"Do you need a hand getting into the tub?"

"I told you to leave me alone, damn it!"

Avy stood, listening outside the door, willing him to get in safely. A grunt, and the sound of sloshing water, assured her that he had successfully lowered himself into the bath. She went to make up the bed and find a fresh pair of pajamas. "Do I dare open the windows to air out this room? Just for a few minutes," she said.

Tea and toast waited for him on the bedside table as Cal, wrapped in a towel, reentered his bedroom. Conflicting emotions erupted: irritation at the cold air blowing in from both windows, reluctant gratitude for the warm nourishment, desire for the welcoming comfort of the freshly made bed, and bewilderment at how it had all been accomplished.

"That Chase woman must have come back," he thought out loud, "but why would she leave the damn windows open?" He hurried into the pajamas and robe laid out on the bed and moved to shut the windows. A woman's rear end protruded from the back seat of the car parked in his driveway. As he muscled the window down, she backed out and turned to look up at him. "Gaelle."

Avy pulled her suitcase from the car and carried, rather than rolled, it hurriedly to the front door and past his sight. He crossed to the other window and struggled to close it before her approaching footsteps reached his room.

"I've got it, Dad. You get into bed and have your toast and tea while it's still warm."

"Don't tell me what to do," he growled.

He blocked her from the window, determined to shut it himself, but it stuck tight. She waited.

"Oh, all right! No sense in letting food get cold. You shut the damn window, since you're the one that left it open."

He stomped back to the bed and climbed in, leaning back against the pillow-cushioned headboard. She watched him pull the tray across his lap, shaking with the effort, then she turned and shoved the window into place. She rested her hands on the ledge and her forehead on the cold windowpane. A sigh escaped her lips and fogged the glass. She was at a loss for what to do.

Chapter 31

Two days later, his fever had passed. Since she hadn't been able to convince him to go to a doctor or urgent care, she wasn't positive, but assumed he was at the tail end of a flu virus. She set him up with hot tea and toast again and left for downtown.

The lawyer had been right. The guardian ad litem had not yet been appointed, let alone the investigation that would allow her to take over guardianship for her father, but something had to happen soon. The situation was out of control, but she had another concern to deal with.

Mrs. Chase was due home that day before noon. Andrew had given Avy a key to the house, and she wanted to be there before his mother arrived. That way she could get her settled and make sure the home care team could provide enough support so Lydia could manage. In the two days recovering from the surgery she had made enough progress that she could walk about twenty-five feet with a walker before needing to sit. Andrew would be staying with her at night in the guest room—his old room—having arranged to trade shifts with another cop who had been bucking for the night shift for the extra pay. The home care nurse was scheduled to arrive in a few hours to evaluate what kind of support Lydia would need during the day.

The empty house still smelled of the last batch of brownies Lydia had made. Avy had found stale remnants of them in an aluminum tin in her father's kitchen. She raised the blinds to an unusually sunny morning for mid-February. Typically, the sky remained a leaden gray for months in winter, leading Michiganders to escape south for some sunlight. But today, it brightened the interior of Lydia's immaculately kept bungalow. Avy knew she would be happy to get back to her cozy home.

She made sure the doorway was wide enough to get a walker indoors, and there was only a one-inch threshold to manage. She wrestled Lydia's overstuffed chair across the room to place it by the picture window and moved a side table and reading lamp beside it. Books lined a bookshelf on the other side. The TV sat on a stand across the room and she angled it toward the chair and set the remote on the side table.

Next, she checked the bathroom. She smiled at the pink furnishings and thought that Lydia must have redecorated after Mr. Chase died. She would need to use the walker to get in, but that should be okay. Essentials were reachable, but she didn't find any medications in the medicine cabinet. That was worrisome.

The bedroom was as she remembered, pale blue with white trim and a white chenille bedspread over the double bed. If necessary, she determined, the bed could be moved against the far wall to make room for the walker or a bedside table. She found a weekly pill-minder on the dresser. It showed she'd been faithful in taking them; until the day she'd fallen unconscious, the slots were empty. Avy opened the next slot. From what she could tell, the pills were baby aspirin, Lisinopril, calcium, a daily multivitamin and two others she didn't recognize. So Lydia was being treated for high blood pressure and the calcium and vitamin showed she was being proactive about staying healthy. She couldn't have prevented the tumor, though.

Avy hesitated at the door to Andrew's old room, then turned away and entered the kitchen. It was spotless, if outdated, just as she remembered it. She found a garbage bag under the sink and removed most of what was in the fridge—after nearly a week Avy didn't want to do the open-and-smell test—milk, bacon, hotdogs, bread (she could see creeping bread mold through the wrapper), cream, mushy-looking blueberries. She left the eggs and butter, as well as condiments that were still under the expiration date, and started a grocery list. Then she checked the freezer and the cabinets. She was moving some essential items to lower shelves when she heard the front door open.

Lydia, head turbaned in white gauze, bumped across the threshold in a wheelchair propelled by a muscular EMT. "Oof," she said, then, brightly, "Avy!"

Her speech was back. "Welcome home, Lydia! I've been trying to make things comfortable for you."

"Are you her daughter?" a second EMT—this one female— asked, following with a walker and a blue hospital bag holding her belongings.

"I'm an old friend. I promised her son I'd be here to settle her in. I'll make sure she's got some lunch and anything else she needs."

"Great. Here are her discharge instructions," the woman said. The male EMT was helping Lydia transfer from the wheelchair to the chair Avy had placed by the window. She checked him out from the corner of her eye while she took the bag and the papers from the other one. Then the woman turned to Lydia. "Are you okay, Mrs. Chase? Shall I put your walker by your chair?" Turning to Avy, she said, "You should be close by when she needs to get up.

She's learned to transfer from a chair, but this one's a bit cushy and she may need a hand."

"We'll do fine," Avy replied. "I'm a nurse." She made a mental note to purchase risers for the chair legs.

"So, we'll leave you in good hands, Mrs. Chase," the hunky EMT said before turning to wink at Avy. They said their goodbyes and walked out the door. Avy hesitated closing it, watching them leave, till they were back in the van.

"He's really quite luscious," she murmured to herself.

As the van left the driveway, Lydia spoke. "Thank you, Avy. It's good to be home." Her words were measured and deliberate.

"What can I get you for lunch?" Avy asked. "There's not a lot in the fridge. I threw most of it out, and I'm going to the store later to replenish what you need. But I could make you a cheese omelet if that sounds good. And a cup of tea? Coffee?"

Lydia closed her eyes, smiled, and nodded. "Tea, omelet, and then a nap."

While Lydia slept, Avy checked with Alliance to see if the nurse was on schedule. She had plenty of time to run to the store. She returned with groceries and a bouquet of flowers and settled everything in place. She checked that Lydia was still asleep and plunked down in the chair by the window when a car pulled up.

A petite young woman bounced out of the car, landing on the driveway in rainbow-colored clogs. She stopped to exchange her winter coat for a white jacket and clipped on an ID badge. Avy watched from the window as the woman slammed the car door and strode to the back of the car. She popped the trunk and disappeared inside, reappearing with a large tote bag and an armload of folders. Avy got up and opened the door to usher her inside.

"Hi!" the woman chirped. "I'm Monica, a nurse with Alliance Homecare. Is this the home of Lydia Chase?"

"It is," Avy said. "Come in." Monica stomped the slush off her shoes on the welcome mat and stepped over the threshold.

"I'm Avy, a friend helping Lydia get settled. She's taking a nap, but I can get her up."

Monica slipped out of the clogs, leaving them dripping on the rug in the foyer. "Perfect!" she exclaimed. "I need to see how she manages getting up and down, so let's just begin with that."

She slipped a newspaper out of the side pocket of her tote and surveyed the living room furniture. "I'll just set this down on the coffee table," she said, moving aside the flowers Avy had placed there and dropping her tote bag on top of the paper. The flower vase shook, threatening to spill. Avy rescued it and carried it with her as she led the nurse into the bedroom.

"Lydia," she said softly, "the nurse is here." Lydia opened her eyes and pushed the light cover to the side.

"Hello, Mrs. Chase," bubbled Monica, pushing past Avy. My name's Monica. I'm here to get things started with your home care needs."

"I'm Lydia. Let me get up."

"Fabulous! I need to see if you can do that without any help, okay?"

Lydia nodded and began the slow process of sliding her legs over the side of the bed while sitting up. She used the walker Avy had placed at the bedside as scaffolding to pull herself up and out of bed. Both she and Avy let out a breath and smiled.

"Wonderful!" Monica exclaimed. "That was perfect! Can you walk, now, to the bathroom?"

Lydia straightened her shoulders and took a step. Then another, until she was at the bathroom door. "Need to go," she announced.

"Great! Let's see how you manage that."

Lydia's eyes widened as she realized that the nurse intended to join her. She glanced at Avy, but bravely entered the bathroom followed by Monica, who left the door wide open.

So much for privacy, Avy thought. She stood to the side in the hallway, not wanting to add another pair of eyes to the scene, but could hear everything just fine. From the bathroom, Monica reported that Lydia would need a toilet seat riser to be able to manage getting up on her own, and she called Avy in to lend a hand in helping her off the toilet.

"I really should not be touching her until I get the consent form signed," Monica explained, in a surprisingly quiet whisper. Avy led the way into the living room, where Lydia gratefully sank into her chair and let out a sigh.

———— • ————

After nearly two hours, Monica had finished all the paperwork and explanations, had justified the pill bottles and med box with the information from the hospital, and outlined for Lydia's approval what Monica thought she needed to be safe at home: toilet seat riser, overbed table, fall alert device, and a reacher. And chair risers, Avy added to the list. And Lydia would have a lot of therapy to help her regain functions that had been robbed by the tumor: physical, occupational, speech. And an aide to help her twice a week with showering. Monica turned to Avy and asked, "You set up her kitchen and the living room?" When Avy nodded assent, she exclaimed, "You'd be a great home care nurse! You knew just how to make it easier for her to be independent."

"Well, I *am* a nurse," Avy volunteered. She badly wanted to let this woman know just how much of a nurse she was—she could have been her boss! "In fact I need to leave tomorrow to get back to my job in New York."

"Oh, that's too bad. We need more nurses in home care, and you're a natural!"

Avy couldn't imagine the tedium of all of the paperwork that Monica had done that afternoon, and she guessed there was more waiting for her after she left. No, she was more than ready to get back to that bright office overlooking the mountains.

Chapter 32

It was dark and chilly on Monday morning when Avy woke to Alex's bark. His overgrown claws scratched at her door. Her alarm was set for 5:00 a.m. but her clock read 3:42. It was a good ten-hour drive back to Albany and she needed an early start, but she hadn't planned on *this* early. Her head fell back on the pillow, but Alex continued his barrage at her door. With a groan, she climbed out of bed, wincing as her bare feet hit the cold floor. She padded across the room. When she drew open the bedroom door, the dog bounded in and threw himself at her bare legs.

"Ow! Hang on a sec, buddy! Let me get some clothes on." Alex whined and circled her legs while she pulled on her sweatshirt, joggers, and slippers, nearly tripping over the frantic dog. "Dad!" she called, but noted his empty bed as she passed his open door.

Alex raced ahead of her down the stairs and through the living room, scratching furiously at the front door. When she opened it he tumbled out, watered his plants, and vaulted back in. She caught him at the door to wipe off his muddy feet, but he wriggled free and bolted for the kitchen.

Avy clambered to her feet. "Dad!" she called again. "Where are you? Alex was in a panic to get outside." No response. A balloon of frustration expanded in her chest.

"He can't have left the house, not when I need to get on the road! I don't have time to track him down."

She followed Alex into the kitchen, hoping her father was asleep at the table or scrounging in the refrigerator. But the kitchen was empty, too. Alex faced her, prancing at the open door to the basement, and the balloon of anger deflated, punctured by alarm. Before she reached the dog at the opening, she already imagined her father's body—crumpled at the bottom of the stairs.

She flipped the light switch but the stairs remained dark. Without hesitation, she grabbed the handrail and scuttled down after the dog. The image in her mind materialized dimly at the bottom. "Shit! Shit! Shit!" Her usual expletives had failed her.

Avy knelt on the cold cement, shoved the frantic dog aside, and shook her father's inert form, shouting, "Dad! Dad! Are you okay?" He remained as motionless as Annie, the CPR mannequin. She felt for a carotid pulse. His skin is so cold, she thought, but there it is—thready, but even. His chest rose as she laid a shaky hand on his pale sternum, between the folds of the unbuttoned pajama top. She rolled him gently onto his side, carefully arranging his legs in a rescue position, and heard him moan.

"It'll be okay, Dad!" She turned to the dog and ordered, "Stay here, Alex. Keep him warm."

Her phone was still upstairs on the bedside table. She hauled herself up to the kitchen, two stairs at a time, then pounded up the steps to the bedroom.

Phone in one hand, she punched in 911, then tore the comforter from her bed as she headed back the way she had come. An ingrained authority took over as she reawakened her expertise as a medical professional in charge of triage. Her steady voice told the dispatcher, "I found my father at the foot of the basement stairs a few minutes ago. He's unconscious and very cold, but breathing. He's probably got some broken bones. The door to the house is unlocked. The basement stairs are just beyond the kitchen which you can see from the front door. I'll be down there with him. You should know that the light to the basement doesn't work so it'll be dark, and there's a friendly dog that may try to get under your feet, so be careful on the stairs."

For a change, Alex had obeyed her, staying close to his master, licking his face. Avy covered her father with the comforter. "Dad, I've called 911. They should be here any minute. You're going to be okay."

Twenty minutes later, following the ambulance to the hospital, she realized she would have to delay her return to Saint Catherine's to sort things out once again for her father.

"Mugwort!" she cried out, pounding her fist on the steering wheel. She wondered if the hospital would grant a short leave.

Chapter 33

One week's unpaid leave was all they offered. If she could not return to her duties full-time by then, she would be replaced. The second-choice candidate, the HR director warned, was an employee of Saint Catherine's and could take over with minimal orientation.

Four days into her leave, her father remained in the hospital with a sacral fracture and three broken ribs. An initial MRI had confirmed a brain bleed, now resolved. But in addition, the hospital neurologist had seen something more. From the MRI and her father's symptoms, as well as consultation with Dr. Nanninga, he diagnosed frontotemporal dementia of the behavior variant type. She didn't recall the term from her training or work in the ICU, so she searched the hospital's medical library and discovered that bvFTD fit his symptoms perfectly. Unfortunately, there was no cure and he would become progressively worse. At least now, she thought, I know what I'm dealing with. But the thought gave her no relief.

The discharge plan the social worker had discussed with her and the guardian ad litem—the GAL—finally assigned, was to send her father to a skilled nursing facility for rehab and potentially permanent placement. She agreed it was the only solution. The GAL was a heavyset man, clearly overworked, who had not even met her father yet. He readily agreed to let Avy take on the responsibility of choosing between the three available SNF openings he gave her.

She walked through the front door of the first place on her list to find patients lined up in the lobby in their wheelchairs, some sleeping with their chins on their chests, others staring vacantly. Not an attendant in sight as she waited at the unmanned reception desk. She pinged the tinny call bell five times.

Her face squinched involuntarily at the acrid smell. The lobby began closing in around her and her hand flew to her chest. She felt like she was back in the dark attic with its smells of mouse droppings and mold. She stumbled out the door as the receptionist finally shambled in. Over her shoulder she called back that she would not be staying for the tour.

"One down. Two to go."

The second facility seemed more promising, as she sat in the sunny waiting room. The receptionist seemed a bit harried and asked her to wait while she attended to a family member. She had no interest in eavesdropping, but his angry voice carried easily despite the woman's efforts to quiet him.

"Can you please follow me into the conference room?" the receptionist pleaded. "I'll have our manager come to speak with you."

"No! I won't spend any more time in here than I have to. We should have been informed of the safety violations before now. And not one, but *three* suspicious deaths? This is outrageous! I'll be removing my mother today. And you can tell your manager he can expect to hear from my lawyer!"

He turned away and, over an armload of clothes, noticed Avy rooted in her seat across the lobby. "If you care about your family member, I'd get them out of this deathtrap!" The receptionist flinched as if physically struck by his words, but Avy nodded briskly at the man, stood, and hustled out after him.

This left her with one option, a converted convent in a downtown neighborhood. The palatial stone building sat back from the street on several acres and looked like a men's dormitory from Cambridge or Harvard in the 1950s. Oaks lined the brick walkway that led to the expansive stairway at the entrance. Snow glistened in the evergreens and on the roof of a gazebo. Avy took in a deep breath and shook the tension from her shoulders. She let a trickle of hope eddy into her chest with the next breath and straightened her spine. She crossed beneath a concrete archway laden with dormant vines of ivy and rang the bell beside the double oak doors. It was soon opened by a middle-aged woman in a simple dress suit who ushered her into the foyer. Dimly lit and quiet, it spoke of old-world austerity and stability, in harmony with its former service.

"Welcome. You must be Miss Lehrer."

Avy took the woman's outstretched hand, smiling in return. "I am. Thank you for meeting with me on such short notice."

"Happy to oblige. I'm Sister Jean, the matron." She handed Avy a colorful folder. "Let me show you our facility."

They left the foyer through a glass door that opened with the matron's badge. Here, the convent ambience vanished. Lighting was much warmer, the hallways spacious, and the furnishings modern and streamlined. Avy could hear unhurried footsteps on the tile floor.

"This is our therapy suite," the sister said, holding open the door to a brightly lit room full of equipment where two therapists worked with an elderly woman. Supported in a sling attached to the ceiling, she took hesitant steps while holding on to parallel bars. The therapists praised her with each tiny step.

They rounded a corner into a patient unit. A large window allowed Avy to observe well-groomed ladies sitting at a table in a common room, working at a craft that kept them in deep concentration. Sister Jean led her farther down the wide hall and stopped at the counter, where she spoke quietly to a woman in white scrubs, who directed them to a patient room.

"All our rooms are double-occupancy," the sister explained as they reached the patient room, "but we do our best to match our residents with appropriate roommates." Avy doubted there could possibly be an appropriate roommate for her father.

She noted that the furnishings were sparse, without much space for personal items, but the room smelled fresh in the light coming through a sizable window, and both beds were made up with colorful spreads and pillows. Sturdy hooks on the wall held a folded walker. Another door led to a shared bathroom.

"It's like a dorm suite. Not much different from mine at the Denver School of Nursing."

"So you're a nurse? That will be a big help in your mother's care, to have a knowledgeable family member involved."

"Oh, it's not my mother I need a place for. It's my father."

As the matron turned to face her, Avy saw that the wrinkles in the matron's face had drawn into each other; her mouth pursed in dismay. "Oh, dear. I think there's been some miscommunication. We accept only *women* here at the Center."

Back out on the street, Avy stood defeated. Her car waited at the curb beside a city park where pigeons waddled, looking for tidbits of anything left behind. Starlings and sparrows darted among them. A few wooden benches were occupied by heavily bundled-up inhabitants. At a distance, the snow-blanketed playground was empty of children.

Dejected, Avy finally pulled her keys out of her jacket pocket and a business card fell out. She picked it up. It was the card the homeless woman had given her. She stood between her car and the park bench where they had sat together. The church rose across the street. Above the doorway, three winged figures looked down benignly.

She thought, why not go in? It might be locked, but she couldn't bear to go home with no solution to her dilemma. If the church was open, she could sit in quiet privacy and try to come up with a new plan. She had three days. The GAL would be no help in that short a time, and she wasn't about to jeopardize her position at Saint Catherine's.

She crossed the street and stopped before the bayberry hedge separating the church from the sidewalk. Pedestrians adjusted their path around her as she stood there.

"Excuse me," called a stroller mom, dashing after an older boy. The woman's elbow nudged Avy out of her inertia, and she moved toward the steps. Mindlessly counting them as she ascended, she reached the top on seven. It would be silly to go back now, she thought, but if it's locked . . . She clasped the brass handle, cold in her palm, opened the weighty door, and stepped into the dark narthex.

Immediately, the smell of wax, whether of lit candles or furniture polish—she wasn't sure—brought back visions of the sparsely adorned Bible church her family had left years ago. But the sanctuary she observed through a transparent barrier of glass was starkly different. Imposing in its height and breadth, it had cream-colored walls that contrasted with the deep brown wood trim of the choir stall. Ranks of organ pipes nearly reached the ceiling. Clerestory windows let light fall into the vast space without reaching down to the pews. Below them, stained-glass windows displayed scenes of Jesus' miracles, spilling a kaleidoscope of colors across the marble floor.

Avy tiptoed to an aisle on the left of the central glass, slipped inside, and slid into the back pew. Her heartbeat pulsed in her chest so hard she felt it might almost be audible in the silent space. She sat in shadow, beyond the range of the opalescent light slanting into the right side of the church through a near stained-glass window—Jesus, standing with men in a fishing boat, holding out his hands across a stormy sky. She recalled the story, and some of the other miracles depicted in the windows on both sides, but it had been years since she had thought about them. When her mother succumbed to the cancer, Avy buried in a bottom drawer the children's picture Bible that her mother had given her, along with any childish faith in miracles.

"Hey, Jesus, I could use a miracle right now," she said, challenging the luminous figure. The church remained silent, no flash of celestial light, no rushing wind, no still small voice.

Yeah, she thought, I guess it's still up to me, then.

"I don't want to disturb you, but please, is there anything I can do for you?"

If the pew had not been bolted to the floor, it would have tipped over as Avy sprang to her feet.

"I'm so sorry! Obviously, I *have* disturbed you," the woman said. "Please forgive me. I was just leaving my office when I saw you slip in." She moved with the grace of a dancer to face Avy from beside the next pew. "My name is Claire and I'm on the counseling staff here. I seem to mistakenly assume that people are here to see me, when they may simply want to be alone for a while with God. Please, feel free to sit and stay as long as you wish." She held her right hand out, palm facing Avy, inviting her to resume her seat.

Avy cocked her head, squinting in the dim light, to examine Claire's face—flawless cinnamon-colored skin, glossy black hair with a few gray sprinkles groomed into a short Afro puff, coffee-and-cream eyes topped with long black lashes, and gleaming white teeth between ripe berry lips. "I've seen you before," she blurted.

"Well, I've been here for a long time." Her lips lifted in a smile that flowed into her eyes. "But I'm sorry. I don't recall meeting you."

"No—we didn't actually meet. I mean I saw you from across the street."

Claire raised her eyebrows, tilted her head, and waited. Avy's knees unlocked and she lowered herself back onto the pew.

"Well, there was this odd woman who hears voices. She told me you're a psychic, although I think she must have meant a psychologist? If I remember right, her name was Josie."

"Ah, Josie!" Claire's face brightened with delight. "Did she have her cat with her? I've never seen her without it."

"Sitting on top of the garbage bags in her shopping cart."

Claire settled into the pew in front of Avy and swiveled to face her.

"I'm not a psychic, or a psychologist, though she may have given you that impression." She smiled. "Part of Trinity Church's mission is to help people in need. I'm the program coordinator. I talk to whoever comes here for help and try to sort out what their needs are: food, shelter, freedom from addiction. Sometimes I do individual counseling."

Avy nodded. "She told me you helped her get her teeth fixed, and that she's slept here before."

"Josie hasn't been here in a while, so I'm glad to hear she's alright."

Avy didn't really consider Josie to be alright, but guessed it was all in one's perspective.

"She said she caught 'afro-sclerosis' from you," Avy volunteered with a tentative upturn of her mouth.

Claire laughed in full-throated delight. "I love her frankness! She's made no secret that she's more than a bit suspicious of my race."

Avy held up the small worn rectangle. "She gave me one of your cards. She thought I needed it, I guess," she said with a shrug.

"And do you?" Claire waited in stillness, her open posture an invitation.

"I don't know." Avy shrugged. "Why would I?" She tucked the card back in her pocket.

"People come to me for different reasons," Claire answered, "but I don't believe you came here today to see *me*."

"No. I was at the nursing facility down the block. When I got back to my car, I noticed it was parked right by the bench where I'd met Josie the last time I was there—I'd been up all night trying to sort some things out, and I guess when she said something about hearing voices, I said that I was hearing voices too."

Claire's body shifted, right elbow leaning on the back of the hard pew, right leg bent beneath her.

"I didn't mean it literally," Avy hurried to explain, "but I suppose she took it that way. I just meant that I was struggling to figure some things out and getting different responses from people that made me question myself. Then I found an old journal of my mother's and learned some things that had me really confused." She gulped in another breath. "But today, everything I tried to do failed, so I decided to come in here for the quiet, to try to sort it all out and maybe come up with a new solution. That seems to be my full-time job lately."

Avy's eyes, lucent as sun-splashed water flowing over a river bottom, met the inviting coffee-and-cream-colored eyes of the woman in the bench in front of her. The tears she'd been holding back found a release, slipping down her cheeks. Claire passed her a packet of tissues.

Avy dabbed at her tears. "My father has FTD—and I don't mean the flower delivery service. It stands for frontotemporal dementia. The other day he must have thought he was walking into the bathroom beside the kitchen, but it was the door to the basement. He fell down the stairs, broke three ribs and his sacrum—fortunately not a hip—and sustained a brain injury. He's in the hospital now. The brain bleed has resolved so they're going to release him soon in spite of the pain from the fractures and his increased confusion, but I can't find a decent nursing facility that can take him. In two days I have to drive back to New York or I'll lose my job."

"Hmm. You've taken on a heavy load. Is there anyone who can share that load with you?"

"My mother died when I was twelve." She ticked her index fingers together. "My older sister has no interest in helping our father—he wasn't exactly kind to us." Middle finger. "My younger brother has just begun a prelaw program in Chicago." Ring finger. "That's all the family I have." Both hands fanned out. "I had hired a home care agency when I left for my new job eight weeks ago, but my father was so obnoxious that they quit. And I can't imagine he would be any better with a different agency."

Her mind turned to Andrew and Lydia. "A friend of mine arranged for his mom to help, but she was just diagnosed with a brain tumor and had surgery. Her son found her unconscious a couple weeks ago and she's just come out of the hospital with home care coming in to help." She paused before going on in a subdued voice: "I can't get out of my head that caring for my Dad might have been too much pressure and exacerbated the symptoms of the brain tumor." Her throat spasmed and choked down any further litany of woes.

Claire's next question took her by surprise—backtracking to the first revelation she had shared with Claire. "May I be so bold as to ask about your mother? She died when you were just an adolescent?"

It had been ten years since she'd spoken of her mother's death with anyone, she realized. Like the release her mother seemed to find in her journaling, perhaps it would help to unburden herself of the grief she'd carried alone for so long. The woman sitting before her seemed prepared to accept it. Avy shifted in her seat, took a deep breath, and began.

"Mom had cancer. I heard the hospice nurse say cervical cancer, but that's all I knew at the time. I was young. I guess they were trying to spare us kids. I've since tried to research it, but I don't know what type she had—if it was hereditary or not, or if it metastasized from somewhere. I'll be starting some screening once I turn thirty. Anyway, even though Mom went through chemo, it didn't help. She just got sicker and . . ." Her voice drifted off into the memory.

"She died at home?" Claire's words gently brought her back to the present.

"Yeah. Hospice caregivers came to our house to help take care of her." The memories were prying their way out from the dark corner of her mind that she had locked, like the snap of the clasps on the old suitcase of her mother's few belongings. "I missed the nurses and the other staff after my mother died; they were so kind to us kids. They wanted to see us afterward for grief counseling, but my father turned down the offer—for himself and us. We just had to pick up and go on."

Claire nodded.

"Maybe I had it the easiest." Avy sighed. "By taking on the care of my little brother, I think I tried to enter into Mom's life. I tried to think of what she would do and how she would act. I don't think it occurred to me at the time, but maybe I thought that if I could become more like her I wouldn't miss her so much."

"It's an interesting coping mechanism, but that seems like a big responsibility for a twelve-year-old."

"My father tried to manage us kids, I guess, but Jared was only three years old." Her brow creased. "And Dad was busy teaching at GRSU so there was only so much he could do."

"You took on your mother's role, then. I wonder how she would handle the situation you're in right now."

"She loved Dad. She'd take him home and care for him." Avy gasped and quickly slammed a mental door on the implication. No, she thought. This wasn't the same thing. She had her own life now and she didn't owe him anything.

She held her eyes open wide to prevent the tears from coursing down her cheeks again and focused on the piercing eyes of the stained-glass Jesus in the boat.

"Don't look at me like that!" she ordered him. She lowered her gaze to Claire.

"I did just sort of ask Jesus for a miracle," she admitted with a scowl. "Although maybe it was more of a challenge than a prayer." Her index finger lifted past Claire's face to land on the face of the stained-glass fisherman gazing down on her. Claire swiveled, her shoulders twisting to glance back at the window.

"But I didn't get one." Avy's hand dropped to the back of the pew in front of her as Claire faced her again. She sighed audibly in the silent space. "It seems it's always up to me to manage things, and I don't know what I can do to fix this mess."

"I wonder if perhaps Jesus *did* hear you and has turned your challenge back to you—if you may be the miracle you're looking for. If that's the case, I think you'll find a way."

Her? A miracle? Avy's skeptical eyes leapt from the gentle eyes of the woman before her to those of Jesus and back again. She felt herself drowning in those matching pools of compassion and understanding.

Doubts and misgivings squeezed her chest and erupted from her throat in an unexpected sob. The colors of the stained glass blurred, forming an iridescent aura around Claire's figure, who moved to sit beside her now, to wrap her in her arms.

Part 2

Chapter 34

She *might* be what Claire suggested—a miracle—but she sure didn't feel like it. What was a miracle supposed to do, or *be*, anyway?

The hospital reluctantly kept her father on the neuro unit longer than they would have liked. Since there was no appropriate rehab facility for him, they had no choice. But finally he was released into her charge along with medications for pain and an order for outpatient physical therapy.

Dorothy Henderson, at Saint Catherine's, said she regretted Avy's decision to remain in Berndtbridge, but they would be offering the position to their internal candidate. Dispirited, she thanked Dorothy for the opportunity and resigned—her position and her freedom—to stay in Berndtbridge and try to manage her father's life. She wondered if she would ever again have a chance to pursue her dream—but that, too, would take a miracle.

For now, she simply needed to earn a living. The words of Lydia's ditzy nurse kept repeating in her head, "We need more nurses! You'd be a natural!"

What a comedown that would be from what she was leaving behind. But working as a home care nurse, she realized, could allow her the flexibility to check on her father at least once each day, between clients, and still make it home by evening when he became most confused and belligerent. With misgivings, she joined Alliance Homecare.

To further her humiliation, she found that Monica, Lydia's nurse, was assigned to be her mentor. They were polar opposites— Avy focused and private, Monica scatterbrained and ebullient. Avy had held her tongue and submitted to Monica's inane instructions. A thirty-day orientation was policy, and Avy *did* respect policy, even if she could have wished for one better adapted to a person with her considerable credentials and experience.

She could be running the place, she grumbled, instead of slogging along in an entry-level position. It was absurd, she felt, for someone with her expertise to have to endure the condescension of a woman who didn't even have the drive to advance herself beyond the rudimentary skills of the job. Monica might be several years older, Avy concluded, given that she had a husband and two kids, but she might have started her family right out of high school, like so many insecure females, making her Avy's junior.

Monica drove her crazy with her childish prattling. Avy's pairing with her had been just one more frustration to deal with on top of everything else with her father and absent siblings, but she was well practiced in masking her emotions. She doubted that Monica suspected, since she now treated Avy like her new best friend. And she was a hugger. Avy shuddered.

Her father had refused any further therapy and seemed resigned to—if not grateful for—her presence in his house. It was time to see if this experiment would work.

By now, Avy had been with Alliance Homecare in Berndtbridge for just over a month and her orientation was over. At least she was on her own now, relieved to be finished with Monica's hovering, and she would face today's frustrations as she preferred—alone.

At Saint Stephen's in Denver, she had never really been alone, yet she had been able to keep everyone at arm's length. She didn't understand why she couldn't have done that again with her father. Instead, she had given up a prestigious job in Albany, a new life on her own terms. She had reached her highest goal, the mountain's summit. But here she was back in Berndtbridge, where the highest elevation was a local bunny hill that felt a lot like her new job. Her bold career path had turned into a dead end, and her newly reclaimed loyalty to herself had lasted a mere eight weeks. Reluctantly, she'd assumed an old, familiar identity—the dependable daughter and caregiver to a recalcitrant father. She didn't feel much like an ethereal miracle—more like a martyr drawn into the gravitational pull of earthbound inevitability.

The subterfuge of mid-March, sunny and pleasant one day, with pelting hail and blustery winds the next, was indicative of her days. She could never count on a day of smooth sailing no matter how well she had planned. And now, it was turning into one of *those* days.

Her face scrunched in annoyance. As much as she had yearned to be independent of Monica, today she could have used her help. The day was crammed. With the phone call last evening, she learned she had to readjust her schedule of homebound client visits to fit in a new admission. The agency's census had dropped as the weather began to improve, and the nurses were expected to take every referral that came in to boost it back up again. She knew the reality of the adage "Last hired, first fired" and agreed to take on Mr. Frederick Hutchins. She added the admission visit to the end of her day and headed out. It would have been a very full day if all had gone according to plan. But, of course, all had *not* gone according to plan.

It had *begun* all right. There was little traffic on the highway when she started out at 7:00 a.m. to drive an hour south to see Agnes, alone in her dilapidated farmhouse by the dairy. To her surprise, she found that she enjoyed the scenery—even in the monochrome of mid-March—while she directed her Focus from one home to another. As she pulled up to the farm, she waved to Agnes' son overseeing the milking of the last row of cows in the dairy barn. She turned and stepped gingerly onto the sidewalk leading to the back door. It was pockmarked with frozen boot prints from the March snowfall followed by overnight plummeting temperatures.

The farmhouse was a museum of odd collectibles gathered over years. She ducked under dozens of cobwebbed kerosene lanterns hanging from the porch ceiling and navigated through grime-encrusted five-gallon glass jugs full of marbles just to reach the kitchen door. It opened only with a jerk to loosen it from the swollen threshold and continued to vibrate under her hand. She made her way over the curling linoleum tiles through the kitchen—cluttered with various eclectic elephant statues, rows of vintage salt-and-pepper shakers, and shelves of commemorative porcelain thimbles—to reach the old woman in her "living-turned-bedroom," where at least fifteen antique clocks kept separate time—or none at all.

Blind and extremely hard of hearing, Agnes greeted her weekly arrival with a frightened, "Who is it? I have a gun!"

After checking the woman's blood sugar and vital signs, making sure there were no bedsores, and examining the log that her son kept of the week's medications and any concerns, she jotted her own findings in the log and headed back up the highway to "pleasantly confused" Mrs. Cairn.

Eloise Cairn's medications were a mess again. As Avy reset the med box, she explained—yet again—that Eloise needed to take *all* her pills, *every* day, from the *box*, not the *bottles*. The woman didn't seem to be suffering any symptoms of heart failure, so Avy figured that, somehow, she must be getting her meds right most of the time, although it was impossible to be sure. She didn't want to have to start counting the pills left in the bottles, too, but that would be the next step. She cupped her hand around her mouth to project the sound directly into Mr. Cairn's ear, and reiterated, "Make sure she takes her pills *only* from the med box, *not* the bottles." The old man, who was deaf but pretended not to be, scowled. "You don't have to yell at me! I can hear you."

Both he and his wife nodded in agreement to her instructions, just as they had three days earlier. She crossed her fingers that her next trip to the elderly couple would prove to be more satisfactory. She really did want them to succeed and remain in their home.

Francis Kohl (Avy's mind always added, "a merry old soul") held a fist to his chest and tried to belch. His angina was clearly causing pain, but he had waited for her to arrive. He was *not* merry.

"You were supposed to be here over an hour ago!" he said, his usually jocular face shriveled up like a walnut shell. She gave him another nitro from his stash, called 911, and stayed to monitor his vitals, hoping she wouldn't have to administer CPR. Much as she liked him, she didn't relish pressing her mouth against his.

Later, when the ambulance siren faded away, bypassing the crawling traffic to speed Mr. Kohl to Berndtbridge Memorial Hospital, her muscles relaxed. She called the office on her mobile to have them alert the hospital liaison while she tried to nose her way out of his driveway onto the busy street to head to her next patient.

He was probably already at the ER, she thought, and she was still stuck there in his driveway.

A gray-pony-tailed black man on a Harley narrowly missed her bumper as he shot through the opening between her car and the stalled traffic. He grinned in her direction and waved as he roared by, eagle wings boldly emblazoned on the back of his worn leather jacket.

───── ◆ ─────

Even the usually routine visit with Camilla was quirky. Her intravenous central line looked fine, and her daughter Janelle was handling her care needs, but she was worried.

"She's just not peeing today," Janelle reported. "There's been nothing in the catheter bag since I changed it when she woke up this morning." A quick check confirmed Avy's suspicions. The clamp was still closed on the tubing, blocking the flow, and preventing the poor woman's bladder from emptying. She opened the clamp and clear yellow liquid poured into the bag.

She rushed through the rest of the visit—vitals, physical exam, IV-line site care, med-check.

One more to go, she thought. Then back to Dad.

It was past 3:00 when Avy pulled up to a two-story yellow house on the corner of Crawford and Bates and cut the engine. A worn sofa sat on the sloping front porch. A stained mattress leaned against the side of the house. The shades in every window on the first floor were drawn and it looked as though the front door was held in place by an assortment of locks. She checked the address in her patient folder. It was correct. The skin on the nape of her neck began to prickle.

"Toadflax!" she muttered. "This must be what a dog feels like when it senses danger." The feeling of skin pores closing into an invisible shield crept over her body. She took a deep breath, patted her lab coat pocket for her pepper spray, and stepped out of the car. At the top of the porch stairs she rapped on the front door and hoped no one would answer.

The last of the four dead bolts clicked. A young Latino dressed only in jeans hanging dangerously low on his hips studied her— long enough for her to note the array of obscene tattoos covering his chest, arms, and face. She was grateful for her Alliance Homecare name tag and white lab coat that proclaimed her as a professional with a nonthreatening purpose, but her hand gripped the pepper spray in her pocket. Finally, he tipped his head toward the stairway. "Upstairs. End of the hall," he said. Avy passed through a gauntlet of hostile stares from the other inhabitants of the crack house and picked her way up the stairs littered with dried dog poop. At least she *hoped* it was dog poop.

At the top she looked back with unease at the front door, as the locks clicked back into place. The nerves in her temples tingled and her ears strained for any sounds beyond the blood she felt rushing through the tiny capillaries in her brain. All was quiet behind the closed doors lining the long, darkened hallway.

She had felt this same hypervigilance when, at age ten, she found herself locked inside another building one Saturday afternoon.

Saturdays held a blessed change in routine from her busy school days. She was allowed to sleep till 9:00 if she wished, but she had a list of chores to accomplish before she could escape the house. When the weather was fine, she spent Saturday afternoons exploring the forested nature center, watching for the appearance of the first spring wildflowers—the spring beauties—or the return of the green herons to their island nest. But she always left enough time to bike to the library before it closed at 5:00. On rainy or wintry days, she spent hours there exploring the world through books.

Avy entered the kitchen that Saturday morning to announce that she had finished her chores, and she overheard her mother's voice complaining uncharacteristically to her father. She had received a call to attend an emergency board meeting at the library at 3:30, "on a Saturday, of all things!" Avy heard only part of the conversation, but caught the words "can't tolerate that kind of behavior from a board member."

Along with Berndt's Bridge and the nineteenth-century township post office, the library was one of several historic buildings in their town. Her mother was an engaged member of the preservation board, so her complaint reflected the cancellation of her afternoon plans rather than an unwillingness to support the community.

Avy arrived at the library, with shoes mucky from tracking a garter snake into the soft mud of the spring ice melt. No one was at the high front desk on the main floor. Before she was tall enough to see over the edge, she used to stand by her mother's side with her nose to the wood, inhaling the rich aroma of linseed oil on walnut. Her fingers would trace the deeply carved molding below the marble edge of the countertop, carefully avoiding the hardened wads of bubblegum plastered there.

Now that she was old enough to check out her own books she preferred to find a spot on the second floor, where she had discovered Judy Blume and Paula Danziger in the Young Adult section. Her mother's meeting was already in session in the conference room. She didn't bother to eavesdrop, but bounded up the granite stairway.

The second floor emitted the ambience of a place for serious readers like herself. Heavy wooden shelves that towered above her head intersected the space and smelled of dust and old leather— like her Grandpa Birk's barn in Iowa, but without the manure. Pyramid-shaped mica lamps swayed almost imperceptibly from the ceiling on long chains filled with cobwebs. The lofty ceiling itself was supported by dark wooden beams that curved down where wall and ceiling met, descending down opposite sides of the room, to form buttresses. Between the buttresses, low bookshelves lined the walls, and windows stretched from Avy's chest almost to the ceiling.

Avy had to use a step stool to reach Judy Blume's *Are You There God? It's Me, Margaret* from the top row of the seven-foot-high shelves angling diagonally from the windows to the center aisle. Then she rolled the metal stool to her favorite window and clambered onto the top of the shelf to settle in till the meeting was over and she could catch a ride with her mother.

In the fading light from her hideaway, she looked up from the final sentence, closed the book, and rested back against the solid buttress for a moment. She rolled her head contentedly to the right to look out at the new leaf buds on the sugar maples below her. The shadows of the young branches played across the library window.

It's so peaceful here, she thought. And quiet.

Too quiet, she suddenly realized. She swung her legs over the edge of the bookshelf and pushed off. The thud of her mud-caked gym shoes hitting the hardwood floor echoed to the ceiling. She took a few cautious steps. Several rows over, the floor squeaked. She froze, teetering on tiptoe, arms spread like wings to maintain her equilibrium, breath stilled. The bookshelves loomed over her in the dim light like cliffs.

What time is it? she wondered. She couldn't see the huge library clock from where she stood, but she guessed by the shadows and the silence that the library was now closed and empty. Empty, except for whatever might be waiting down the other aisle.

She tiptoed to the end of the row and peeked into the wide center passageway. Nothing. But the openings to the aisles between the bookshelves loomed, like dark cave mouths, between her and the stairs. She was positive that in one of those dark clefts lurked a terrible something poised to attack her. The clock ticked in the silence just out of her sight. Her temples throbbed. Are you there, God? It's me, Avy, she prayed. She had to get out of there! Something— God?—nudged her from behind and she bolted for the stairs.

She had reached the landing at the turn of the steps when she heard a sound below her—a key in the lock of the heavy front door. It swung open and a voice called, "Aviana! Are you here?" She raced down the stairs and flew into her mother's arms.

———— ◦ ————

But here, at the top of the crack house stairs, her mother wouldn't appear with a key to unlock all those locks. *God* wasn't there pushing her out of danger, either. Taut muscles in her temples pulled her glasses tight against the bridge of her nose, bringing her myopic focus fractionally closer as if she were pulling an invisible shield around her body. She inched down the dim hallway, holding her breath as she crept past each silent door. In her sweaty left hand, she clutched her heavy nursing bag, ready to use it as a weapon if necessary. Her right hand gripped the pepper spray, thumb ready on the pump trigger. At the end of the hallway she eased back slowly on her heels, flexing and releasing her tight calves. She took a few slow, deep breaths, and knocked.

The sound of muttered curses, bed springs squeaking, and unsteady footsteps preceded a fumbled rattling at the doorknob. She stepped back as the door opened inward and sudden sunlight outlined a huge form looming in the doorframe—her library nightmare in the flesh.

"Who d'you think *you* are?" he bellowed. The grizzled drunk faced her in the doorway, feet planted wide apart for balance, and blinked in her face through a filthy mat of hair.

"I'm your miracle," she blurted out, and wondered where that had come from. "I'm the one who's supposed to keep your toes attached to your foot and your foot attached to your leg," she said. "You can let me in and cooperate or you can throw me out and lose it all—and probably your life along with it. It's your choice."

"Yer my *miracle*? What th' hell's that supposed to mean? You gonna wave yer magic wand and—'poof'—my foot's as good as new? Ought t'ave jus' cut it off an' be done with it," he grumbled. "I s'pose that meddling little social worker sent you here," he sneered, "like she threatened t'do when I lef' the hospital." Avy flinched as he bent his muscled, six-foot-four frame over her and fingered her name tag with fissured nails. His breath was as foul as she'd ever inhaled, foul with alcohol and rotten teeth. For a moment the man wore her father's face.

"So yer Aviana, huh? What you got in your little black bag? Any presents for me?" She realized the wisdom of never carrying narcotics, syringes, and needles into a patient's home—and why nurses carry pepper spray. Her hand gripped the canister in her pocket. Just say the word, she breathed, and I'm out of here, shaking the dog poop off my shoes. She longed to write, "refused services" across his chart.

He stumbled back, waving her in with an unsteady, sweeping bow. She eased past him, feeling the doorframe scrape across her shoulder blades, pain shooting down her spine.

"Mind if I set my bag down? It's heavy." Avy pointed toward the unmade bed. She pulled a newspaper from the outside pocket of her bag to act as a shield between it and God-knows-what vermin might be crawling in the sheets. She had already picked up head lice from a patient and had no desire to repeat that fiasco. As she remembered the incident, her scalp began to itch and she fought the urge to scratch.

"Leave the door open, please," she ordered before he could swing it shut. "It's a little close in here." Even with the window wide open in this weather, she thought. She told herself that a quick escape route was more important than confidentiality. The stench of urine pervaded the room. Not again, she thought. It would cling to her clothes, her car. She'd carry it back home with her. She wondered if anyone ever flushed a toilet in this place, and hoped she could get out of there without barfing and adding that scent to the lovely mélange of aromas.

He shrugged and left the door standing wide. Staggering back across the littered room, he flopped into a legless, oatmeal-colored armchair by the bed. Without even looking at her, he reached out his hand. "Gimme the papers. I know the routine. You people never do nothin' without me signin' away my gonads." Impatiently he copied his shaky signature, 'Fred Hutchins,' six times, before she could explain what any of the forms were for.

Great, she thought, a frequent flyer.

"Let's get this over with." Grimacing, he pulled the stiff brogue boot off of his bare foot. A dry coppery stain showing a green patina spread across the thick gauze wrapping his toes.

"Before we take off that bandage, I should have the Betadine soak ready so we can set your foot right in it. They sent supplies home with you from the ER?"

"In th' bag over there under th' table." He waved in the general direction of the open window.

Her shoes stuck to the floor, and as she stooped to pick up the bag full of sterile supplies, her face hovered over a pink hospital basin on the table. A dead fly floated in a bath of cloudy urine.

She had always managed to keep the delicate structure of her professional persona from collapsing by preparing for any possible threats to her stability: Icy pavement? Take your time and watch your step. Medication chaos? Reinstruct and reorganize. Heart attack? 911, Nitro, and monitor. Lack of urine output? Check catheter and open clamp. Traffic? Count to ten and breathe. Each threat to her well-ordered plan had caused her carefully assembled structure to wobble, but she'd held it together by force of will—until now. She couldn't have foreseen how this assignment would lay siege to her defenses, eroding her composure.

She fell apart. She wheeled on Fred, yelling, "You pee in a *basin*? That's supposed to be for soaking your foot! What's the problem with using a *toilet*?"

"Hey, Missy, you woun't use it either if you saw it. The people who live in this dump"—he bellowed into the dark hallway—"you don' know what you might pick up from that toilet." A loud cackle sounded from behind a door down the dark hallway.

He lurched out of the chair and stumbled to the table, shoving her aside. He grabbed the basin and flung the urine out the open window. It splattered on the yellow mound of dirty snow below. "Happy?" he asked, slamming the basin back down. Droplets leapt up, spattering her lab coat. He limped painfully back to the chair. "Get on with it!"

Black Swallow-wort, her brain cried. That was so unprofessional! She scrambled to pick up the pieces of her competent persona. Cleaning the basin with water and hand sanitizer would demonstrate her determination and give her time to calm down and think. So she squared her shoulders and braved the putrid bathroom to return the basin to its intended purpose. Clearly, she realized, she wouldn't be able to bully Fred into compliance, but still she would give him her best care, regardless of the disgusting environment. She was a professional! She returned with the warm-water-and-Betadine soak and set it down on the floor at his feet. Maybe, she thought, she could pull off a good outcome out of this impossible situation, like a magician's parlor trick. She would try to work her magic—if only she *did* have that wand—to heal up his infected toes and save his foot.

"Okay, Fred, let's get on with it." She needed to get home to her father.

Growling and yipping resounded from the darkened house—like a terrier flushing a fox from its hole—as soon as Avy opened her car door. She held the leaking bag of Chinese food at arm's length over the grass while she leveraged herself out of the car and ran for the kitchen door.

"Hey, Dad! You okay?" she shouted, rushing the dripping mess over to the sink. "What's with the dog?"

"He's a flaming nuisance, that's what!" His angry voice came from the laundry room. Alexander the Great snarled. At twelve years he still had all of his teeth and knew how to use them. She hoped it was just a trimming session that was causing all the snarling—from both individuals—behind the closed door. Alex was not supposed to shed, but unless he was trimmed to within a finger's breadth of his skin, his hair found its way into every nook and cranny of the house. She had even found it in her mouth at dinner one night.

"Would you like some help?" she called. The more hands anchoring the dog's wriggling legs, the better. Patience had never been a strong suit for her father. More often than not, she remembered, Alex came out from under the clippers looking more like an overgrown rat than an aristocratic hunting dog.

"What I would like regarding this beast you don't want to hear."

It must be one of his good days, she thought, and chuckled.

"But, yes, of course I would like some help! Don't let him out the door when you come in or he'll steal that Hunan chicken before you know it."

So, she thought, he still recognizes the scent of his favorite Chinese dish. The longer she was in the house, the more she remembered her father's preferences. By catering to them, she tried to avoid his outbursts.

"It's safely dripping in the sink," she said.

"I still wouldn't put it past him," her father growled as she slipped through the door. Alex nearly wriggled out of his grasp before she caught his haunches. "Shthupid mutt." Her father picked a clump of white fluff off his tongue as she took over.

"I know what a pain he is."

"He's an unmitigated nuisance!" Then, as Avy gently scissored the wispy hair on Alex's ears, her father reached over and scratched the dog's chin. "But Jared loves him." His voice had calmed as he spoke of his boy. The two of them worked together silently, Avy clipping, her father playing with the dog's ears.

The sun had set by the time she nuked the chicken.

Chapter 35

Nick Katsoukas was as chiseled and handsome as the marble bust of Hermes in her father's study. Like the Greek god, he had pallid skin that was smooth and cool to the touch. But unlike the mythical messenger, Nick barely spoke. Avy coaxed whispered answers from his blistered lips in order to obtain the minimum information she needed to admit him to care. She often resorted to yes-and-no questions to avoid inducing pain in his ulcerated throat. In the week since, she had seen him every day, along with his aged landlady, Tilda Berndt, who made up for his reticence. Each day when Avy finished her quiet hour with Nick in his expansive upper-floor apartment, the old woman was found lingering in the foyer at the bottom of the staircase. Massaging her arthritic fingers, she would ask, "How is he today? Any better?"

"Tilda, you know I can't discuss Nick's health with you. It's private. Just like I couldn't tell Nick anything if you were my patient," she reminded her.

"Oh, I wouldn't mind at all," she assured Avy. "He's such a nice young man, and I know he'd be just as concerned about me as I am about him."

"Well, I can tell you that he appreciates your concern and that the soup was just what he needed. Here's your container." She smiled, placed the greasy Tupperware in Tilda's hands to put a stop to her inquiries, and pivoted to the door, but she was arrested by Tilda's voice continuing. She couldn't bring herself to be blatantly rude to the woman. Resigned, she turned back to listen despite her own wish to be alone with her thoughts in the privacy of her car.

The office had called her just before she arrived at her appointment with Nick to tell her that the jovial Francis Kohl, the merry old soul whom she'd grown to enjoy, had died the night before from a full-blown heart attack. Though he had called 911 this time, he was deemed DOA when the EMTs brought him into the emergency room. His niece called the office to inform them of his death. She wanted the agency, and especially Avy, to know how much he had appreciated being able to stay in his home and that he had been very fond of his nurse. Avy wanted the solace of slowing down and marking his passage and her loss, but Tilda had other plans.

"I don't know how I would manage this house without those boys," the old woman said, absently setting the Tupperware on the console table. "I can't climb those narrow stairs anymore since I broke my hip. That was the year before Mr. Berndt passed. I haven't been down to the basement or up to the second floor at all, but those two have gladly helped with whatever I need. It's made it possible for me to stay here where Louis and I lived our whole life together."

Avy's eyes followed Tilda's gesture encompassing the quaint, high-ceilinged living room. The furnishings spoke of bygone comfort and refinement: faded floral silk armchairs and matching camelback sofa, Persian rugs, a spiraled mahogany stair rail and moldings, an eight-person dining set in the glassed breakfront, and a Baldwin grand piano.

"I have so many memories here, and such beautiful things that my husband bought for me when he traveled out of town for his work." Her wistful voice spread a gauzy veil of memories over the room. Avy voiced her appreciation with a murmured "mmhmm," and turned toward the door, but Tilda wasn't finished.

"And my garden." Tilda turned to gaze out the picture window at the crocuses and daffodils pushing up out of the soil. April had brought buds on the twigs of several trees. "We planted that birch tree when we first moved in, and apple trees in the back. Every year on our anniversary, Louis would find a new tree or flower to add." She paused, a wistful smile drawing her wrinkled skin upward. "But I couldn't keep it up these last few years. Then Nicholas arrived like an answer to prayer. He knows so much about gardening. It's never looked better since the boys moved in last year about this time."

Avy seized the opportunity of Tilda's reverie to reach again for the doorknob. Too late. The old woman turned from the window with unusual energy.

"Jessie's been badgering me to sell the place. She insists it's not safe for me to live here anymore, but I can't leave my home. It was her home, too! She loved this house when she was a girl. Louis made her a Victorian dollhouse to match this one. It was so big, he had to build it right in the room upstairs—the apartment the boys are in now. It was her playroom until she decided she was old enough to have her own apartment and we moved her whole bedroom up there." Avy had heard snippets of this before. Jessie was Tilda's daughter who lived in another state.

Tilda's shoulders hitched up mischievously and her eyes danced. "So I hatched a plan that would stop her nagging. I hand-lettered a nice sign—I can do calligraphy. Did I tell you? Well, I will admit"—she paused, rubbing at her misshapen fingers—"the lettering is a little shakier since Arthur Itis came to stay. Anyway, I hung my sign on the wrought iron fence out front, right beside my Duchess of Sutherland rosebush—Louis planted it for me just before he passed. The sign advertised for an upstairs boarder to help with the chores."

"That very evening"—she giggled, and her cheeks pinked up—"this handsome young man was riding by on his bicycle, just like I saw him do every day, morning and evening. He always admired my garden. If I was outside he would call out 'hello' and wave as if I were a young lady he was flirting with. It was quite exciting, actually, the high point of my day."

"Well," she laid her hand over Avy's on the doorknob and leaned in conspiratorially, "that day I happened to be indoors when he appeared, but from the front room I watched him admire my garden as usual and smile his beautiful smile as he rode by. Then suddenly he turned his bike around in the middle of the street." She jerked her petite body to the left with surprising alacrity, holding imaginary handlebars as she always did at this point in the story. Avy's hand was wrested from the doorknob, gripped firmly in Tilda's. "He pedaled back and jumped off his bike to read my sign. Then he looked up at the house and waved at me!"

That was how Nick, a lab tech at Berndtbridge Memorial downtown, had settled into Mrs. Berndt's life and home. He and his friend, an architect named Nate who lived in a cramped loft in the arts district, had decided to pool resources and find a place with both room and character, near enough that Nick could bike to work. He enjoyed puttering outdoors, something he had missed in his fourth-floor apartment. And according to Tilda, Nate was proficient at every sort of home project.

"I thank the good Lord in heaven every day for those two. They're like sons to me—or maybe I should say grandsons. Only now I worry so about Nicholas. He does seem to get sick a lot." She paused finally, giving Avy the opening to let slip the information the crafty old lady craved.

Avy again reached surreptitiously for the crystal doorknob, and Tilda repeated her daily invitation. "May I offer you some tea, dear?" Last week Avy had once been swayed by the charm of the antique-strewn front room to accept Tilda's invitation, stepping back in time while the old woman plied her for details about Nick's health. That's when she learned that Tilda's husband, Louis, was descended from the original founder of the town, a wealthy lumber baron. In 1869 he had built the covered bridge that spanned the river, allowing him to build his home on the east side and his lumberyard on the west side, where the current floated the logs right to the sawmill, down from the forests up north. The lumberyard was long gone, but the house was the same one Tilda still occupied. From the lumber baron and his bridge, the town got its name.

Normally Avy declined the offer of tea, but this morning her heart was heavy with Frances Kohl's unexpected death and Nick's aggressive illness. She succumbed to the comfort of hot tea the disarmingly persistent woman offered. She sank into the overstuffed armchair and let her head fall back on the hand-tatted antimacassar—a new word she had picked up from Tilda when she had referred to it as a doily the previous week. Warm sunlight bathed her face and seeped into her chest as she let her eyelids close over the welling tears.

She wondered if she had done the right thing in enabling Francis to stay at home; had she made the right decision? Maybe he'd still be alive if he had moved into the assisted living facility like she'd recommended in the beginning. And what about her father? Should she have found a nursing home in some other location, like

Albany? Could she have managed to keep her position at Saint Catherine's and taken care of his needs as well?

Second-guessing changed nothing and only wracked her with uncertainty and regret. In this work, most of her patients were as old and likely to die as Francis Kohl or even Tilda here. Not like Nick, who was only a few years her senior. She gratefully accepted the hot tea, the brief respite from death, and the one-sided conversation of her hostess.

Chapter 36

Weeks ago, she had asked her new client the routine opening question, "What goals do you hope to achieve with help from home care?"

"To dance at Orli's wedding," was the petite lady's unusual response. "That is all that I wish for." Her stubborn eyes had locked on Avy's startled ones, as if daring the nurse to deny her this ambitious goal.

"When is this wedding?" she had asked, stalling her response. Abigail told her the chasuna, the Jewish marriage ceremony for her granddaughter, would be held in late spring, seven weeks after the Jewish Passover that was just celebrated.

"Seven weeks is not a long time." Avy hedged. "When the physical and occupational therapists come, you can work out some short-term goals to start on, but I don't see how we can have you dancing in just seven weeks." The elderly woman snorted and fixed her with an unblinking gaze. The challenge was on.

Avy smiled, recalling that first encounter. Abigail Rosenberg—three days poststroke—had sat, propped in a damask armchair, a cross-stitched pillow supporting her flaccid right arm. Her slender hands rested gracefully in her lap, her unadorned right held loosely in the bejeweled left. Gold-slippered feet crossed daintily, left over right, at the ankles. The satin robe, royal blue edging the pale concavity in her chest, revealed a gold chain and a diamond drop pendant nestled against her throat. Only a faint downturn of the right corner of her mouth and a drooping of her right eyelid from Sunday's stroke remained on her delicate face. Her speech and her flashing eyes were untouched. As were her faith and her stubborn determination.

"The Scripture says 'there is a time to mourn and a time to dance.' I am done with mourning over this injury to my brain. I will *dance* at Orli's wedding," she insisted as Avy stood to leave that day.

She's obviously a pampered old matriarch used to getting what she wants, Avy thought. When it doesn't work out this time, I wonder how she'll feel about God.

She had informed Ryan, the physical therapist, and Shannon, the occupational therapist, of Mrs. Rosenberg's conviction. Ryan called the next day, after his evaluation, and confirmed her judgment. "I've been proven wrong before, but there's no way she can meet that goal in just a few weeks. I'll be lucky to have her on a quad cane by then."

Avy fell into scheduling these visits before going to see Fred in the smelly crack house, to fill her senses with beauty and to avoid carrying Fred's essence into the lovely home. Abigail Rosenberg lived in private quarters in the luxurious house of her daughter Devorah and son-in-law Samuel Weismann, prominent members of the large Orthodox Jewish community in neighboring Cascade Village.

Passing by the mezuzah on the doorpost on her weekly visits, she entered a different world each Tuesday. The Italian marble foyer of the house opened onto a cathedral-ceilinged living room in muted taupe with mahogany and silver accents. A massive floor-to-ceiling display case, glassed in on both sides, separated the living and dining areas. It displayed an eclectic collection of menorahs, silver spice boxes, and kiddush cups from Israel and other parts of the world.

Grace, the Jamaican maid, welcomed her at the door that day. She led her, as always, down the marble hallway to the right, swaying to an inaudible rhythm. Avy's own body picked up the gentle rhythm as she followed through another mezuzah-adorned doorway and into Mrs. Rosenberg's apartment. Grace called softly, "Miss Abigail, ma'am, the nurse is here."

"Thank you, Grace. Please bring Aviana a glass of ice water, would you? With lemon, yes?" Her ritual of refreshment.

She had warmed toward Mrs. Rosenberg over the weeks. She was gracious and kind, not at all the spoiled matriarch she had originally thought. And the woman had a clever sense of humor that she employed in her persistence to have things turn out the way she wished. She had even attempted to convince Avy that she must be Jewish, Aviana being a Hebrew name, she insisted. "It would be translated as 'God my father answered' or 'God is my father.'" When Avy assured her that her father's line was German for several centuries and her mother's line was Dutch and Irish back to the twelfth century, Mrs. Rosenberg raised her eyebrows. "My dear, Jews have lived in every corner of the globe for centuries! You may be unaware of the Irish Jews, but surely you've heard of their presence in Germany."

Avy reddened. She realized she'd made a stupid blunder. Abigail took pity on her, lightly switched tacks, and began referring to her as a "good Christian girl—like Grace."

"Christian, I guess, and maybe I used to be a good Christian girl," she said, "but I'm not—"

There was a soft knock on the door and it opened a few inches. A striking ginger-haired girl, looking decidedly Irish herself, peeked around the edge.

"Bubbe," she said, "I don't want to interrupt, but I'm going shopping and wondered if you needed anything."

"Motek shelee!" Abigail cried. "Come in! Come in my sweet!" The girl complied and swept in with a bright smile. "Aviana, this is my lovely granddaughter, Orli. Orli, meet Aviana, a good Christian girl, and my wonderful nurse." She winked at Avy, who swallowed her useless protest and acknowledged the young woman with a gracious smile herself.

Orli reached her grandmother and bent lovingly over her, kissing her left cheek. Abigail caught her chin in her hand as she straightened.

"What! The other cheek you don't like?"

The girl laughed, bent down again and gave the right cheek a resounding smooch. Avy noticed she wore a simply tailored midnight-blue dress that appeared cool despite the long sleeves. A matching silk scarf held her hair back and accentuated her deep blue eyes and the sculpted cheekbones she had inherited from her "bubbe."

"Thank you for the good care you're giving my grandmother," she said, turning to Avy. "She's working very hard with the thera-pists, and Grace and I do the exercises with her, too. If God wills it, she says she will dance at my wedding."

"From your mouth to God's ears," Abigail interjected before Avy could cast doubt.

Her granddaughter smiled lovingly at the old woman. "Omeyn," Orli responded, waved goodbye, and shut the door softly behind her.

She wished Ryan's prediction could be wrong, but he held little hope. Nor did she.

"So, you want to know how I'm progressing, yes?" Abigail asked, after Avy had listened to her heart and lungs, checked her blood pressure and pulse, and taken her temperature.

"I have no pain—God be praised. My bowels and bladder are working fine. My appetite is quite good. No headaches, blurred vision, or ringing in my ears. Every hour I shift my weight and I have no sore spots on my tush." She grinned as she finished the recitation.

"Nothing wrong with your memory either! I don't even have to ask the questions anymore!"

"But more importantly, look at this," she demanded. She reached a trembling right hand across her lap to pluck a narrow book from between the seat cushion and the left arm of the chair. She opened it to a ribbon-marked page.

"You *are* a good Christian girl and you should appreciate this," she announced, arching her left eyebrow to show she would brook no argument. She read aloud, "'I know nothing, except what everyone knows—if there when Grace dances, I should dance.' One of your poets wrote this."

"W. H. Auden, yes." Brit Lit was one of Avy's favorite subjects in her senior year of high school, and she knew that, in Auden's poem, "Whitsunday in Kirchstetten," the line followed a more somber sentiment about how to act in a catastrophe. So, maybe it was fitting. Abigail had suffered a catastrophe, and her choice was to dance. Auden would be pleased.

"You're right, yes! Now," Abigail continued, with dancing eyes. "You've met Grace. She will be accompanying me to Orli's wedding, and she will most assuredly be dancing. She cannot help herself! So, I will be there when Grace dances, and Auden says I should dance! Who am I to disappoint him?" she finished triumphantly.

Avy shook her head, grinned involuntarily, and rolled her eyes. The woman was incorrigible. "Well, you sure get points for determination," she said, but she needed to bring Abigail back to reality.

"Shannon must be pleased with the progress you're making with your arm strength. Your small motor coordination has really improved, but let's see how that right leg's coming along."

"King Solomon said, 'The end of a matter is better than its beginning, and patience is better than pride,'" she said, forcing her right foot to slide forward a few inches. "So, God knows I have pride. Now I learn patience, yes?"

"From your mouth to God's ears," Avy responded.

"Omeyn!"

Chapter 37

She had offered to cover several of Monica's patients on an unseasonably warm spring day when her colleague was overloaded. She enjoyed seeing someone new and often reveled in a patient's invitation, "You can come back any time Monica's too busy." But Mrs. Dougherty was not one of those.

Eileen Dougherty was in renal failure and was due for a blood draw today. Avy had scheduled her for first thing in the morning, so she could follow up on the lab results before the end of the day. She dreaded patients who were in renal failure; they could be so prickly. She got enough of that from her father, although some days were better than others. She tried to avoid his triggers, but on most days, it was impossible to know why something set him off.

She hadn't counted on Rolf, Mrs. Dougherty's Doberman, who flew at the screen door when she arrived.

"Could you put the dog in another room, please, before I come in?"

"Rolf! Come!" the woman called from somewhere inside. "He's perfectly harmless," she yelled. "What are you waiting for?" Avy entered to find her overstuffed patient settled deep in an equally overstuffed chair in front of the television, the dog's nose resting on her feet under a TV tray. She was sure she heard his throat rumble.

As she set up her equipment for the blood draw, he rose up and hovered around her suspiciously. Then, just as she was inserting the needle into the woman's left antecubital vein, Rolf seized the opportunity to poke his muzzle into her crotch.

The vein blew as she jerked back. She loosened the tourniquet and stanched the bleeding with a gauze pledget, using perhaps more pressure than was actually necessary, while Mrs. Dougherty lashed out at her incompetence.

"Now may I *please* put him in another room?" Avy begged.

"Don't you use Rolf as an excuse for jabbing halfway through my arm!" the woman screeched. "He's here to protect me from stupid people like you who don't know how to do their job! He'll stay right here."

She sighed and prepared the right antecubital site, aware of Rolf's vigilant stance at Mrs. Dougherty's side, his mouth just inches from her hands. After the poke, blood gushed into the tube. She loosened the tourniquet from Mrs. Dougherty's doughy arm, internally satisfied with her wittiness, gently slid the needle out, and again stanched the bleeding with one hand. With her other hand, she deftly slid the blood-filled tube from the vacutainer syringe and set it carefully on the hearth.

"There, you see? Rolf had nothing to do with making you hurt me. Like I said, he's here to protect me!" Avy silently turned to dispose of the needle and syringe in her sharps container, when Rolf seized the blood tube in his slavering mouth and gulped.

Mrs. Dougherty's face turned from pasty to ruddy.

Avy refastened the tourniquet.

A few minutes later she walked out the door with a new blood sample while Mrs. Dougherty furiously dialed the vet.

Monica owed her for this one.

Next on her list was Jack McAlerney, living on the fourth floor of the Riverside Apartments downtown. The building had once housed a Victorian-era brothel, Monica gossiped, but it had closed down in 1910 and remained empty for years. Finally, during the Depression, it was reopened as a boarding house, and later as a hotel. It wore its history like a ragged overcoat. She dragged open the door that led into the run-down apartment building and was engulfed in the smoke of cigarettes, cigars, and possibly something illegal as well. Unable to prevent her nostrils from flaring, she nodded to the residents lined up on chairs against the wall of the dingy foyer, held her breath, and trailed an old woman shuffling, with a rolling walker, into the elevator.

"Five," the woman barked while initiating a slow turn to face the closing doors.

"Got it," Avy said, pressing the button for the fifth floor. "but I'll be getting off at four."

The woman nodded disinterestedly. Avy turned away. She pushed the button for the fourth floor, then the fifth again. The elevator didn't move.

"Hmm. Slow elevator," she mused aloud.

Just then it jerked to a start; the pulleys five floors above them squealed in the shaft. Elevator music would have been nice for once, she thought.

"So. How long have you lived here?" Avy hated small talk—it never really seemed to reduce the awkwardness of a forced closeness—but it helped to diminish the unnerving sounds coming from the antiquated contraption.

No response. She glanced toward the woman, who stared resolutely at the elevator door. Well, almost there, she reasoned. She would definitely be taking the stairs down. She shifted the weight of her bag to ease the pain in her back, which seemed to be getting worse since she had started this job. With the new laptop and all her other supplies, it weighed twelve pounds. Avy faced the buttons and noted that number four was no longer lit. She sprang forward to punch it in again when the floor beneath her fell away. The woman beside her fell forward onto her walker as they plummeted.

"Chicory!" Avy screamed, hitting the threadbare carpet, her shoulder blades crashing down on the walker. Pain sliced through her and she discovered what it felt like for the first time to lose bladder control. *Thank goodness for my heavy periods,* she thought briefly and hoped the pad caught it all. The elevator cage shuddered to a stop.

"Holy Mary, Mother of God," the woman moaned.

Avy disentangled the woman from her walker and propped her against the wall. "Are you alright? Does anything hurt?" She swept her eyes over the fuming face and aged body.

"Jesus, Mary and Joseph!" the woman swore. She grabbed the walker handles, hoisted it overhead, and crashed it against the doors.

"Okay. That answers that question," Avy murmured. She crawled to the emergency phone and lifted it from the wall. Above her, the pulley squealed back into life and they began to rise.

"Get me out of here!" the woman screamed.

"I'm calling for help right now!"

"By the time they get here I'll be buried alive at the bottom!"

"Just try to stay calm and stop beating the doors! We don't want this thing shaking!"

"Otis elevator," a voice droned over the phone. "Are you having an emergency?"

"We're in one of your elevators that just about dropped us to our deaths!"

"Where are you, Ma'am?" The voice had lost its apathy.

"In your death trap of an elevator!"

She covered the mouthpiece. "What's the address here?" The woman didn't look up from the rosary pulsing through her fingers.

"Just a minute." She fought to recall her GPS reading. "It's Riverside Apartments in Berndtbridge." She fell backward, retaining her hold on the phone, as the cage plummeted again.

"Be with us in the hour of our death!" her companion screamed. The elevator lurched to a stop again at the end of her supplication.

Avy righted herself, dragging herself up by the metal phone cord. "Sixteen something southeast on Seminole!" she shouted into the phone, simultaneously sliding the heel of her hand over the buttons for every floor.

"Help is on the way, Ma'am. Just stay calm." The phone went dead.

The pulley was lifting them again. "Keep praying!" she blurted out to the woman, sprawled on the floor beside her.

The cage stopped. A new sound—a benign *ding* like a chime calling them to worship—and a crack opened between the doors. Avy grabbed the walker and wedged one of its legs into the crack near the floor.

"Push!" Avy ordered. The doors ground slowly apart, enough for her to shove the woman and her rosary to safety beneath the legs of the walker. Lighter by a hundred pounds, the cage began to rise again, the doors still held open a foot by the walker. She feared that the walker would get stuck at the next floor and the elevator would drop again. She threw her bag through the opening and slid out behind it to fall beside the woman on the floor. The battered walker was forced out and toppled onto her as the elevator continued to rise.

"Are you two all right?" said a face above her. They had landed back in the dim lobby, interrupting the smokers, who stared with open-eyed interest at the unlikely scene unfolding. "We've had trouble with that elevator before." The old man shook his head sadly.

A uniformed man—a police officer, she surmised, looking at him upside down—ran through the doorway. Andrew?

"Don't move!" he said. But her spunky companion had already righted herself and was beginning to rise with the aid of the mangled walker. Andrew's attention turned to the woman as she brought the wrath of God and all his saints and angels down on the heads of whoever was responsible for trying to kill her.

Avy stood, with the assistance of the old gentleman. He looked at her with concern as she straightened her lab coat, wincing with pain.

"You're not the nurse looking for Jack McAlerney, are you?" he asked solicitously, patting his chest. He hoisted her bag and offered her his arm. She gave Andrew a sheepish grin as Mr. McAlerney led her to the all-purpose room off the lobby, where he set her bag on top of a piano bench and dropped down beside it. "You can check me out right here," he said. "No need to go up to my room."

She vowed to let Monica see Fred the next time *she* needed a day off.

Chapter 38

N ate—that's Nicholas' roommate—he's so intelligent about these things. He researched the proper colors for the time it was built in 1873, and they brought some friends home and did the whole thing in one weekend. Jessie will be pleased, I think."

Avy finally got an opportunity to respond. "I don't know what the house looked like when Jessie was last in town, but she can't help but be pleased." The charming Victorian had been restored to its original glory with a fresh coat of paint—"Fieldstone." The trim was a pale gray, and the doors and shutters stood out in slate blue.

"It's too bad she won't see it with all the flowers in bloom," the old lady mused, setting the fragile teacup back on its saucer and gazing through the original rippled glass of the picture window.

"When is she coming?"

"It's hard to say. She's so busy, you know, as a school superintendent over in Milwaukee. It's difficult for her to get away, but she thinks she can take some time when the school lets out for the summer."

"Well, there should be lots of flowers blooming by then."

"I don't know. The perennial beds, I suppose, but I don't think I'll be able to get many annuals in this year."

Nick had done the spring yard work before he became too ill; he'd trimmed back the perennials to encourage new growth and raked up the last oak leaves that fell after the late snow. Now, he told her, Nate would have to help Mrs. Berndt with planting the annuals. Nick's doctor had forbidden any further work in the garden after his histoplasmosis infection was cleared up. Dr. Altman was sure Nick had inhaled the fungal mycelia from the soil that he loved to work. Coaxing beauty and life out of dirt fed his soul, he told her, but it had wreaked havoc with his body.

In spite of the amphotericin B that was infused daily into his vein, he was still losing weight, his lymph nodes were painful and swollen, and his eyesight had worsened. Now his breathing was becoming rough as well, and Dr. Altman had scheduled a chest X-ray.

Nick had first contracted HIV six years ago. He'd worked as a volunteer phlebotomist and counselor when the free HIV clinic was open on the weekend. One day, he told her, a twenty-something woman barged though the door. She dragged a guy in a black hoody behind her by his sleeve. She didn't even try to control her disgust for her sullen companion, but shoved him down in a plastic orange chair. Nick picked up her paperwork and led her down the hall to his small examining room.

"She told me she found birth control pills in his backpack, with another woman's name on them," he explained while Avy began her routine assessment. "After a browbeating I'm glad not to have witnessed, he confessed that he'd been seeing this woman for months. He was worried about getting the lady pregnant but hadn't even considered the chance of getting an STD." Nick struck his forehead with the free palm of his right hand while the amphotericin B flowed into his left arm. Avy shook her head, concurring with the guy's lack of sense.

"I let her vent while I took the blood sample," Nick continued. "As soon as I slipped the needle out of her vein, though, she pulled her arm back to shake her fist, cussing the guy. It shoved the needle right into my thumb." He flexed it. "They both had HIV. I still hate that guy, maybe as much as she did."

Chapter 39

At the office, Avy craned past Ryan's shoulder to see the screen-saver photo the physical therapist had just uploaded. It was three-year-old Marji, the last of Ryan and Natalie's four children, sitting in her mother's lap on a blanket at the beach. Clothed in a red-and-white-checked romper, she reached both hands toward the camera. A wide grin spread over her mischievous face. From the photo, one couldn't tell she had cerebral palsy. Ryan swiveled his chair to address Avy.

"She's just started hippotherapy," he said.

Avy pulled away from the screen to peer at him, one eyebrow raised. "Okay, I'll bite," she said. "What's hippotherapy?"

"C'mon," he teased. "Your Dad's a classical languages scholar and you can't figure out hippotherapy?" As an undergrad at GRSU, Ryan had to take Latin in preparation for medical school before he switched to physical therapy. Though he had never been one of Professor Lehrer's students, Ryan knew of his reputation. Calvin Lehrer was legendary among the classical language students for high expectations and grueling exams.

"Well, hippo could be 'horse' from the Greek 'hippos,' right? So, what's horse therapy then?"

"You're an animal person, aren't you? Why don't you come out tomorrow and watch Marji's session? I volunteer there on Saturday mornings, working with the bigger kids. The rest of the family comes too. We'll pick you up if you want."

———— ⬧ ————

Ryan's three oldest—Emily, 14; Aynsley, 12; and Brian, 8— smooshed together in the third seat of the van to make room for Marji and Natalie in the middle seats. Avy rode in front with Ryan, but twisted her head and shoulders back for a good part of the trip to hear the kids in the back. As the van wound through the countryside, they popped out of place like ill-fitting puzzle pieces, eager to instruct Avy on their various roles at the therapeutic riding center.

"Emily's allowed to lead the horses, but I'm still a side-walker," Aynsley said.

"Okay," she said, pretending she knew what the girl was talking about, but her face must have shown she didn't.

"A side-walker walks next to the horse to keep the rider from slipping off," Aynsley explained.

"So wait a minute. It takes three people to provide a riding session for one student? A leader, a side-walker, and the therapist?"

"Uh-huh. But not everybody needs a side-walker, and some need *two* side-walkers. Plus, the therapist doesn't walk with the rider, since he—"

"Or she," Emily said.

"Or she," Aynsley continued, "is in charge of up to four riders at a time. And we walk about a mile for each half-hour session. You have to walk really fast to keep up with the horse. And you have to be tall enough to keep a hand on the rider's thigh if they need it to steady them." She sighed. "I *hate* walking with Pete's Pride. He's sixteen hands high! By the end I feel like my arm is permanently stuck over my head!" She executed a right shoulder roll to loosen up in anticipation of the task. "Emily's got the easy job."

"Yeah, right! If he doesn't step on me, or blow snot in my face!" Emily said. "I have to keep my eyes straight ahead to guide the horse," she said, taking up the lesson. "They're trained to go in the direction the leader is looking, and if I slow down the least bit Pete's Pride could be right on top of me. Nobody wants that guy stepping on their heels."

"I wish I could be a side-walker," Brian said from between his sisters. "Soon I'll be as tall as Aynsley, but I'm not old enough. I'm still just grooming the horses and shoveling shit."

"Brian!" Natalie warned.

"Well it is!"

"I don't get it," Avy said. "You pay for this therapy, I suppose, but you all work there, too?"

"Yeah! It's fun!" they chorused.

"Fun!" Marji echoed, limbs flailing in her excitement. Avy couldn't understand how this child who seemed to spasm with every movement could possibly relax on top of a huge animal. It seemed like it would take a dozen hands to keep her safe.

"Ryan gets paid as a therapist, but the rest of us are volunteers. Families aren't required to help out at the stable," Natalie said, "but it's been great for all of us to have a family activity that benefits Marji, and that teaches the kids the satisfaction of volunteering. All of them have gained some self-confidence and compassion. It's been a blessing, a real gift from God."

The van pulled a dust cloud behind it into the gravel lot. The crisp April morning held the sharp animal scents that Avy loved.

Natalie raced the kids to the stable and disappeared inside. Avy was tempted to follow and revel in the smell of sawdust, oiled leather and "horse-doovers," as her little brother used to call the pungent droppings, unlike Brian's more literal description. Instead, she waited for Ryan and Marji. She was curious to know how the therapy worked. Ryan unbuckled Marji, lifted her from the car, and held her gently till her spasms settled. He fastened a tiny riding helmet on her head and they headed for the outdoor arena. A sweet-faced Haflinger pony circled inside the fence, led by a young man in cowboy boots. The chestnut's flaxen mane rippled down her neck as she responded to his soft voice.

"There's no saddle," Avy said. She could see a thick blanketed pad and a strange-looking handle cinched behind the horse's withers.

"Not everyone uses a saddle," Brian said. "That gadget on the horse's back is called a surcingle. The rider holds on to it for balance. For this little girl, the therapeutic benefit comes from the transfer of movement directly from the horse to the child and from the child to the horse. In Marji's case, the horse's gait helps her learn better balance and it loosens up her tight leg muscles. It's like passive range of motion, with the horse doing the work instead of the therapist. Eventually, we hope she'll begin to develop appropriate muscle strength without the spasms."

He sat on the edge of the mounting block, holding Marji. Already she was beginning to rock in rhythm to the approaching horse.

"Look at her!" Avy whispered.

"Yep. It's hard to explain but there's something about these big beasts that moves these kids—both physically and emotionally. The rhythm of the horse transfers to the rider and can improve calm and focus. In riding a horse, they escape the limits of wheelchairs or crutches, or emotional disabilities. They sense an acceptance from the volunteers that assist them as well as from the horse that they ride."

"What did you mean when you said, 'from the child to the horse'?"

"Horses are incredibly empathic. The horse can sense both emotion and physical pressure from the rider and respond to what the child needs. He can even match his heart rate to hers within minutes." Ryan had molded his body around Marji's, unconsciously matching his rhythm to hers, just as he described of the horses. Avy ached to be part of something that nakedly symbiotic. To feel her heart beat in rhythm to another. She recalled fleetingly the loving embrace of her mother's arms around her, of her own young arms around Jared. She felt her body begin to sway and wrapped her arms around her belly.

"I've seen some incredible progress with kids and horses," Ryan was saying, eyes on the chestnut circling toward them. "Sometimes within a few sessions. I worked with a seven-year-old autistic boy. His parents were having a really hard time getting through to him and controlling his impulsive behavior. After a month on Peaches he was humming to her, stroking her neck. Eventually he would talk to her—simple things like 'whoa' and 'good girl' and 'walk on.' That's the phrase they're taught to use when they're ready for the horse to move." Ryan looked over at her, leaning beside him on the rail. "It's not a cure, by any means, but it's something, and it gave his parents some relief."

"Hey, darlin'!" called the young man leading the Haflinger toward the mounting block.

"Look, Marji," Ryan said. "Here comes Mr. Sawyer and Miss Pat."

Bubbles of laughter burst from the little girl.

"Well, don't you look excited!" Pat said, climbing on the mounting block beside Ryan. He set Marji's feet on the block and moved out of the way for Pat to hold her steady. "But we better be

real quiet now so Sawyer can bring Sassy over here." The rhyth-
mic rocking set in again as her horse sidled up to the mounting
block. Pat lifted her up and eased her legs gently apart to hug the
horse's back. Marji unclenched her hands to grasp the surcingle
and looked straight ahead between the horse's ears.

"Okay, honey. What would you like Sassy to do?" Pat asked.

"On!" Marji cried.

"That's right. Walk on please," Pat said, and Sassy stepped
away from the platform into a gentle walking rhythm. Ryan gazed
after his daughter and the team. Then Emily stepped out of the
barn, confidently leading a huge Belgian. Aynsley hustled ahead
of them to the platform, kicking up dust, followed by a tall, older
gentleman in a cowboy hat. Ryan turned to greet a teen walking
stiffly toward them from the parking lot with a walker.

"Hi, CJ! Are you ready to rock 'n' roll?"

"Not Pete's Pride," CJ whined. "It's gonna hurt!"

"Only until you relax," Ryan coaxed. "Then just think how
good you're gonna feel." He plopped a helmet on the boy's head
and thumped it with his knuckles.

"C'mon, CJ," Aynsley joined in. "If I can stand him, so can you!"

The teen snorted like the horse standing in front of him in the
arena as he fastened the chin strap himself. He left his walker at
the base of the stairs, grasped the stair-rail with both hands, and
levered his stiff legs up the three steps to the top of the mounting
block. Pete's Pride eyed him attentively.

"Ready, boss," he said.

Ryan and the older side-walker guided him slowly into the
saddle on the horse's broad back as he winced, eyes squeezed shut.
"We'll wait till you're ready," said Emily.

Aynsley and the other side-walker each rested a hand on CJ's
thighs, providing support as his taut muscles gradually relaxed into

their new position in the saddle. The intense concentration grip-ping his features abated as he settled and opened his eyes. Ryan eased his feet into the stirrups. CJ's back straightened, his eyes focused between the horse's ears.

"Walk on please," he said.

Chapter 40

She still visited Fred at the crack house every other day. Ideally, he should be able to take care of his own wound by now, but even with her professional care, the wounds were at constant risk of infection due to his living situation. And she didn't like to pass him off to anyone else—not even Monica, despite her encounter with the blood-tube-snarfing beast, Rolf, and the killer elevator in Mr. McAlerney's building. She saw Fred on weekends even when it wasn't her turn to work. He trusted her, and the other residents in the house didn't spook her anymore—although her pepper spray remained handy in the pocket of her lab coat, just in case.

She never knew if that situation might change, though—when Fred might be drunk again, or when someone else might throw the front door open. Dealers came and went at all hours, but Fred usually met her at the door now, his massive presence serving as her bodyguard. And he usually saw her out as well. She chose not to disturb that delicate sense of security by introducing another nurse.

Every day, whoever was on the other side of the door would call out, "Who's there?" When it was Fred's voice, she always responded, "Same person as always!"

This morning the dressing smelled ghastly. Her nose wrinkled in disgust and tears gathered in her stinging eyes. The big toe wound looked as if it had been caught in a paper punch and green drainage oozed from it through the dressing and onto his sock. It was impossible to guess which item of filth had penetrated it this time; there were so many possibilities. She had a standing order for a "wound culture as necessary" and always carried a swab kit with her. He may lose this foot yet, she thought, while getting a sample of the putrid goop.

"So, Little Miss Avy, what made you decide to be a nurse?" Fred asked while she gathered the sample.

She was beginning to wonder herself at the wisdom of choosing this profession. She was crouching in a filthy crack house bedroom, afraid to touch anything, bathing the putrid toes of an old drunk who didn't care if they fell off or not. The truth was it was how she could escape from her hateful father and make a better life for herself. But aloud, she muttered, "I wanted to help people."

"Same reason I became a cop," he said.

Startled, she looked up from his bloated foot to his unshaven face.

"You think I'm lyin'. It's true," he insisted. "One of Chicago's Finest here. Should have seen me in my uniform! I patrolled the Magnificent Mile." His yellowed teeth showed dimly through his mustache. "It didn't work out."

She could see that. Her plan hadn't worked out either. "What happened?"

"I got bored." He shrugged. "Greedy. One day I busted a shoplifter and he passed me a diamond necklace and a baggie of crack. So I let 'im go, told my partner he had nothin' on him. Word got around the street that ol' Fred was okay." He chuckled. "It put a little more excitement into the job. Took the force almost three years t' figure out what was goin' on."

She lifted his foot out of the basin and onto a blue pad and began dabbing gently with sterile gauze squares. She wondered if she should believe him.

"Joliet Prison was *not* a friendly place for an ex-cop." His nostrils twitched. "But it toughened me up. Ouch!" He jerked his foot from her grasp. "Damn it! That's tender!"

She dragged his foot back onto the blue pad. "You just said you were tough!" she challenged. "Buck up, flatfoot!"

"Who do you think you are?" His challenge ricocheted down the hallway.

"Same person as always." She packed the gaping hole, now free of green gunk, with iodine-soaked gauze tape, wove clean gauze gently around and between his toes, and pulled a fresh tube sock over the dressing.

Really, who was she after all, she wondered, as she headed to Abigail's home. No, she wasn't the same person anymore. This job, her father—they'd turned her into somebody she wouldn't even have recognized a few months ago.

It was past lunchtime when she left the yellow house, but she wasn't hungry anymore. She tossed the lab coat into the dirty-items-box in her trunk, sprayed room freshener liberally over herself, and pulled her spare coat off the hanger in the back window. As she drove away, she reflected on the small progress she had managed with Fred. If not for her, his foot would certainly have been amputated, and the infection would have spread quickly into his bloodstream and killed him. And she cared about that, now.

Chapter 41

"You remember that I'm going to dance at Orli's wedding, yes?" Abigail asked.

"Were you and your husband dancers?" Avy asked, to avoid a disagreement. "Or did you dance professionally?" She's tiny enough to have been a ballerina, Avy thought, while situating the pediatric blood pressure cuff on her client's arm.

"*All* Jews are dancers, but not the way you're thinking." Abigail smiled, the pressure on her arm did nothing to limit her response. "You've never seen a Jewish dance, no?" she asked.

"Only in the movie *Fiddler on the Roof*," she admitted.

"Ah." Abigail nodded. "So what did you notice about the dancing in the movie that was different from what you are used to?" she asked.

She could think of all kinds of things. That whole world seemed so foreign. She didn't answer and her face reflected hesitation in the furrowed brow and slightly opened mouth. So Abigail continued.

"For us, dance is a joyful expression to celebrate God's goodness, his faithfulness to us as a people, and his blessings. Dancing at a wedding celebration is also a *mitzvah*—a blessing—for the

bride and groom, accepting them as a couple into the fellowship of
the community. It says to them that they belong and their marriage
will be supported. But"—she emphasized with an index finger held
aloft—"the big difference is this—we Orthodox Jews dance sepa-
rately. Men with men. Women with women. To do otherwise is
unseemly. No offense meant."

Men with men. Nick's face materialized behind Avy's eyes.
He had contracted HIV from an infected blood sample, but she
suspected he was gay and could just as likely have been infected
by unprotected sex. In many circles—her own, to be honest—*that*
was unseemly. Now she was hearing that in the orthodox Jewish
custom it was unseemly for a man to dance with a woman, but
not with a man. *Oy vey!* She mentally smacked her forehead as she
realized she was beginning to assimilate to whoever she was with.
Nowhere else would *oy vey* come to mind!

"No offense taken," she said, belatedly. She tried to explain.
"In my father's Christian upbringing, dancing was forbidden, so I
was never allowed and never learned to dance."

How could the Jewish faith, she wondered, which is anchored
in keeping so many strict laws, have room for dancing? The Chris-
tianity she remembered from her childhood outlawed so many
things. Yet it claimed to be based on love rather than law.

"Somehow, even when other religious practices were lost, my
father held on to his taboo of dancing, probably more out of fear
that it would lead to something even *more* unseemly. I can't imagine that my mother would have agreed—she had a way of dancing
even as she walked out in the fields—but she died before it was
an issue for me. I can still hear my father's warning, though." She
raised an eyebrow in imitation of her father, wagged her finger at
Abigail, and intoned, "'Dance is a vertical expression of a hori-
zontal desire.' I always thought that maxim was my father's own

creation, but later I heard that it was George Bernard Shaw who first said it."

"Feh! He must have been a gentile, this George Bernard Shaw," Abigail said, waving away the man's ridiculous prejudice. "He should break his left leg and his right arm!"

Avy burst into laughter and impulsively hugged the old woman. Yet even as she did so, the label "gentile" wormed its way into her brain. Of course, gentile referred to her, too. She could pick up some Yiddish, but she was still an outsider, a gentile, a goy. Looking in. Longing to understand and belong. Wanting to be accepted for herself, not just for how she could support and serve others. Needing—she didn't know what, but the need felt like a large stone in her throat.

Chapter 42

"Please let Nate know he's doing a great job," she said to Nick. He would be on IVs until this infection was cleared up and would have been kept in the hospital if it hadn't been for Nate.

In spite of the side effects of the medication for his fungal infection, Nick Katsoukas was still a stunning specimen of humanity. If anything, his weight loss only clarified the perfect bone structure of his face. The fine lines of his chin were interrupted only marginally by swollen lymph nodes, and he could generally hide beneath his collar the fat deposit—a side effect of his HIV medication—rising on the back of his neck.

The drug took six hours to infuse into his vein. She came at 1:00 every day, prepared the medication, hooked it up to the pump, and observed for any adverse effects for the first half hour. Nate would discontinue it in the evening by 7:30. She'd never met Nick's roommate. He was a busy partner in an architectural firm downtown and was in the office or on-site all day, sometimes even on weekends.

"But he's home each evening between 6:00 and 7:00," Nick reassured her, "and he handles the equipment like a pro. He had to pass the nurse's scrutiny at the hospital before they let me come home."

She—and more importantly, Nick's doctor—approved of the arrangement since Nick, as a lab tech, also knew how to tell if something wasn't quite right with the infusion and could stop it early if need be. She relaxed.

Nick's throat sores had cleared and he could talk without pain now. As he had come to trust her nursing tenderness and her personal respect, he had begun to speak more freely. She spent that Wednesday listening to his story trickle out while the toxic medication dripped into his bloodstream.

"My dad was married to the Navy more than he was to Mom," Nick said as she started the infusion. "I remember moving around a lot when I was little, but by the time I was in fifth grade we had finally settled in San Diego. Dad was stationed out at Point Loma at the U.S. Naval Reserve, and he had high security clearance. I still don't know what he did, but he did it with wholehearted devotion, I can tell you. Nothing was higher priority than his work."

Nick's jaw tightened despite the swelling in his neck. His eyes settled on the drip chamber of his IV infusion.

"At home, everything had to be set, predictable, controlled. I was expected to do what he said without question. He determined what was right for all of us in the family, what would keep us functioning the way a proper family should, so that his work would not be compromised."

The sound of the amphotericin B dropping rhythmically into the drip-chamber punctuated the silence. Avy empathized with Nick's painful memories: At least she had her mother, she thought. She wondered if Nick's mother was as supportive as hers: if she was able to nurture his sense of self.

"I didn't set out to rebel," he said, "but I was really turned off by hearing my friends, ten-year-old kids, brag about wanting to enlist so they could shoot the enemy and blow stuff up. All that macho posturing. What was the point? I just couldn't see myself killing people. I wanted to be a *doctor*—most parents would have been proud! But that wasn't part of the family plan."

"Usually it's the eldest son who rebels, my counselor says, but my brother Stefano marched in lockstep right behind Dad. He enlisted on graduation day, along with his cadre of like-minded guys."

Nick's rheumy eyes followed her gloved hands as she palpated his left arm: no redness, swelling or rash. So far, he was absorbing the medication without any toxic effects that she could see on the surface, but who knew what it might be doing deep inside to his bone marrow and kidneys? They wouldn't know until the damage was done.

"This sounds like other stories I've heard," she said. "Domineering father, lack of love in the home. I've heard it's a setup for turning out gay."

Nick gently stopped her examination of his IV site with his right hand. "It's not that simple," he said. "A lot of the guys in my school had the same family dynamic. San Diego's a big Navy and Air Force town. But, believe me, they weren't gay!" He smiled wryly and leaned back in the recliner.

"I had this great buddy in seventh grade named Kevin," he told her. "Both of us were into environmental stuff even then. We worked together on our seventh-grade science project on how amphibians were affected by pesticides. We got all the way into the state science fair that year. That summer we talked our parents into letting us go to a wilderness camp together. It was the same summer that I rocketed into puberty, and suddenly Kevin was more than a buddy to me, but when we got home from camp he wouldn't have anything to do with me."

Nick began his own examination of the IV tubing.

"Eighth grade was hell," he murmured in monotone. "Suddenly words that I'd heard jokingly tossed about like a jockstrap in the locker room were aimed at me. No matter what I said to deny it, I was labeled, set apart, and tormented. I hated myself for the revolting little slime I thought I had become, but as awful as I felt, I knew it would be a thousand times worse if my father heard about it. So I withdrew from all my former friends and toughed it out to the end of the year. Thank God I went to a big public high school in the fall where I could get lost in the crowd."

Nick had shrunk into his pillow. His thoughts seemed to have drifted back in time. When he spoke again, his voice tore at her heart.

"Can you imagine what it's like to fear, every minute of every day, that the rumors and vitriol will start up again? I avoided guys religiously at the same time I was so attracted to them."

He looked full into her eyes and grinned. "I didn't have the same trouble with chicks. They flocked around me like I was the mama hen. I'd get phone calls late at night. One of them would be in tears because her boyfriend, usually one of the football jocks, had broken up with her in spite of her doing everything he wanted. 'And now what will everyone think?' she'd cry over the phone. So I'd have her hang around with me until her bruised self-esteem healed a bit."

An impish smile tugged his face. "I began to get a reputation as a ladies' man, and I didn't try to set anyone straight—especially my dad! I could handle his lectures about being a gentleman much more easily than his revulsion if he found out the truth."

She could understand the girls' attraction to Nick. Not only did he look like a Greek god. He was sweet and easy to talk to. She'd barely avoided spilling her guts to him—but that would be so unprofessional!

"So how did you and Nate hook up?" she asked.

"That's probably not the best term." His forehead furrowed and his eyelids drooped. "Nate was the miracle that saved me after a whole lot of bad hookups," he responded, then paused. "You sure you want to hear this?"

She nodded—struck by his use of the word "miracle." It rang like the chimes at Trinity Episcopal. Another person referred to as a miracle. Curiosity combined with an unexpected compassion for this vulnerable man. Never, since her mother died, had she been allowed this far into someone's personal life. She was not one to get phone calls in the middle of the night—someone looking for a shoulder to cry on. And she had always believed that her professionalism kept her from being judgmental. But, she had to admit, she'd always thought that AIDS was a punishment for indulging in sick behavior. Men with men. Women with women.

"Okay then. After successfully making it through high school, it was assumed that I'd enlist, just like Stefano. When I admitted that I had already enrolled in the premed program at San Diego State University, my father literally turned his back on me. He stood up from the dinner table without a word and left the room. That evening when I got home from my summer landscaping job, my suitcases were packed and waiting in the front hallway. Mom followed me halfway up the stairs, pleading for me to change my mind." Angry determination flashed across Nick's features, drawing his skin taut as he continued his story.

"I retrieved the one thing I wanted, relieved that no one had found my copy of *The Advocate* hidden under the dresser while dumping my clothes in the suitcase."

"That night I made my first trip down to the Hillcrest District—the gay area in San Diego—feeling as free and as petrified as a thirteen-year-old heading off to summer camp."

Sweat ran into his eyes—a side effect of the infusion. He wiped his forehead with a corner of the pillowcase. She waited for him to continue.

"I didn't have to spend more than a few nights in my car. I was taken in pretty quickly—'fresh meat' as they say. I was pretty lucky at first. I met a guy who was also a student. He steered me clear of trouble for a while, but he dropped out of school and out of sight after my first semester and I was left to pay the rent on our shared apartment or go back to living in my car."

He looked at her appraisingly. "You don't look so hot, girl. Is this too much information?" She felt her face burn, but shook her head. "I don't think we'll go into how I paid the rent that winter," he said.

He continued. "I had started out as premed, but I realized I couldn't afford to go for four years anymore, let alone med school. I lucked into a job as a lab assistant and got enough credits in two years to earn an associate's degree as a lab tech."

"Meanwhile . . ." he glanced at his watch and back at her, resting uncomfortably on the edge of Nate's drafting stool. "You still have a few minutes, girl?"

"My time is yours for another ten minutes," she said. "Then I've got to run."

"Great." He shifted in the recliner and inhaled before resuming.

"Meanwhile, I was enjoying my freedom as a gay man at a time when 'gay pride' and 'gay rights' were the new bywords. I had completely left my former life and hadn't spoken with anyone in my family for two years. Then we started to hear about this strange illness that was affecting only gay men. GRID—Gay Related Infectious Disease."

"What we now know as AIDS. I didn't know it had another name," she said. "That must have been frightening."

"Not really. It was all happening up in San Francisco, so we weren't all that worried. I continued to do whatever I wanted for a long time. I had settled into a pretty good relationship with a guy named Jerry, but we both saw other men too. Working in the lab, I heard rumors that the virus was spreading and that it was passed through contact with blood. Fortunately, my lab training kicked in and I started protecting myself, but I couldn't convince Jerry that it was a serious problem.

"I learned to be much more cautious. I started volunteering at the new AIDS clinic in San Diego, doing both the blood testing and counseling about prevention. That's where I got poked with the needle. When I tested HIV-positive a few months later, Jerry spooked. He decided to get out of California. He figured the risk was lower elsewhere, and headed out east."

Nick sighed. "I was so lonely. I couldn't go back to the indiscriminate hooking up that I'd done before AIDS. Suddenly I had this crazy notion to try to reunite with my family. I drove the ten miles on Saturday morning to the house I hadn't seen since I walked out the front door with my suitcase, my *Advocate*, and my determination.

"A young blond woman, pregnant, knelt in the yard, tugging weeds out of the lush yellow sedum that I had planted eight years before. I watched a little boy shoot back and forth on his Big Wheel. It needs a wheel alignment, I thought, watching the chubby legs pumping. Then he jammed down on the pedals to make it brake and spin around before peddling furiously in the opposite direction." Nick's face softened momentarily.

"Watching these strangers who so obviously belonged there, I wondered, how could my folks have sold the house? The woman had seen me pull up with my car windows rolled down, and I had stopped at the curb near her child. She stood up from her kneeling pad and took a few steps in my direction as I reached for the stick to shift my old Ford Escort into first.

"Then, over her shoulder, I saw the same kitchen curtains that I remembered, fly apart, and my mother's astonished face pressed up to the window." Nick's right hand lifted from the chair arm, reaching with longing into a distant memory. "She yelled for my father. 'Ari! Ari!' I could hear her excitement through the closed window of the summer-sealed house. 'It's Nikolai! Nikolai is outside!'"

His arm fell back, but his eyes still stared beyond her, sitting at his side.

"The blond woman looked at my mother, then back at me, perplexed, and stood still in the grass. Her son continued to throw himself into pedaling nowhere, oblivious to the drama of the prodigal's return." His eyes smiled briefly.

"My father wasn't about to prepare a fatted calf for me, but he didn't stop me from walking through the door while he retreated to the hallway threshold. Mom threw her arms around me and held on. I could feel her shaking. Finally, she broke away but still held on to my hands as if I might disappear. She introduced me to my brother's wife who had come up behind us. She had enticed her son Brandon from his Big Wheel with the promise of a popsicle, and followed me into the house.

"Mom explained that because Stefano was out at sea so much on the cruiser *Horne*, Dad had decided it was better for Pam and Brandon to live in the family house." Nick began reciting in an older man's voice: "'She'll have company and can help mother keep up the place.' The last time Pam had seen Stefano was when he was home on leave after Operation Desert Storm. So that meant my niece- or nephew-to-be must be about five months along, I figured. Then both the women went quiet and retreated to the kitchen for the promised popsicle, leaving me and my father standing silently, face-to-face, in the living room." Nick paused, took a deep breath, blew it out, and continued.

"I don't know why I thought I could come back," Nick said, rolling his head against the back of the chair. "Mom and Pam fixed a nice lunch and we tried to make small talk over Dad's silence, but all the time I knew it was time to tell them who I really was."

"This time I didn't exit quietly. When I dropped the g-bomb, Pam snatched Brandon from my lap and ran upstairs. My father rose, just as he had eight years ago. This time he didn't turn his back and walk out. He reached across the corner of the table, pulled me up by my shirtfront, and smashed his fist in my face." Nick's fingers clutched the armrest.

"I could hear Mom screaming through the rushing sound in my ears and my father yelling obscenities at me—his *son*. I had never heard him swear before, but he made up for it that day."

It was more than side-effect-sweat moisture running down Nick's face, and the rivulets on her cheeks were a match for his own. "You have no idea what it's like to feel such rejection, such a complete void of any love, understanding, or hope for reconciliation in the future."

The tears running down her face were not just for him. Yes, they were triggered by his story, but they sprang from that dark place that had settled in her own soul the day she'd left home. She thought, no, she couldn't fully understand his pain. She had so little room for it.

"You're sweet, Avy, and I'm sorry I've made you cry," he said, taking her hand, still encased in a sterile glove. It was hard to feel love and compassion through latex. Maybe that's why they don't like to use condoms—the random thought leaping, unbidden, into her mind. She was horrified at her own stereotyping, still, and wiped her face with her sleeve to hide her eyes.

"That all happened years ago. I was unsuccessful in killing myself that night, so I decided to follow Jerry to Michigan and see if we could make things work. It really hurt that he was not happy to see me—he refused even to introduce me to the gay scene here, but I found my way in anyway. Right away, I found work at Memorial, and within a few years helped to start the AIDS clinic here in town.

"I met Nate one evening—Hey," he squeezed the hand he was still holding. "Pay attention now. I'm about to finally answer your question!" She forced a smile.

"I met Nate when I was doing a seminar on safe sex at the clinic. He was this big, earnest-looking, clean-cut, college-grad type—the kind I love to see in my presentations, because they hang on my every word!" He grinned. Her continued effort to smile supportively was molding her face into hard plastic, but Nick didn't seem to notice. He was engrossed in the more recent, upbeat part of his story.

"In fact, I watched him at the break, and he picked up all the materials we had out on the table in the back. But he seemed reluctant to talk to anyone, so I caught him after the presentation. We went out to talk over coffee and we've been together ever since." He opened his hands, tipped his head to the side, and smiled up into her downcast face.

"See? Happy ending!"

She opened a two-pack of sterile gauze four-by-fours, handed him one, and they both wiped their damp faces. Nick's "happy ending" was not the end, though. He had entered a new phase in his illness and she was afraid the ending would be far from happy.

Chapter 43

It was already 2:45 when Avy finally gave in and asked for directions to the house of her last patient of the day. Bernard Ten-Haven hadn't answered the phone when she tried calling an hour ago or she would have gotten directions from him. But Osmer was a small town—didn't even have a name on the highway exit sign. Avy assumed that by just driving down Main Street she would hit the cross street that he lived on. Instead, she had wasted fifteen minutes driving around, past the Post Office (closed), the VFW Hall (also closed) and the bar (open). The radio signals bounced back and forth, depending on the direction and altitude of her car, between her favorite eclectic music station, WYCE, and WJOS, a local gospel music station. The GPS was worthless. It showed her driving through empty fields since she had left the highway, and kept telling her to return to the highlighted route. She slapped it off, widened her search and passed a row of propane tanks painted to look like cows. She had found TenHaven Lumberyard, but the gate in the chain-link fence was locked and no one answered to her shout or her beeping horn.

She drove back nearly to the highway exit before spying a
pair of jeans stretched out under an apple tree by a farm stand.
It was still cool for the beginning of May, but sunny. Warm
enough to enjoy lying in the grass if you had the time. The sign
by the road read "Kryst Produce" and listed "potaters—5/$1.00,
aspergrass—$1.00/bunch, cow crops—corn, oats, wheat." Beside
the mounded produce a coffee can accepted "cash only" and
warned "GOD IS WATCHING YOU."

"Sure, I know where old TenHaven lives," the kid under the tree
said, rising up on scrawny elbows. "What do you want him for?"

She pulled a damp dollar bill out of her lab coat pocket. "I'll
take a bunch of your asparagus," she said, enunciating the word,
"and I'd be very grateful if you would tell me how to find his house."

He gathered himself up slowly, mischievous eyes never leaving
hers. He was young—maybe still high-school-aged—if he even
went to school. "Sure I can't interest you in some of this year's oats,
too?" he drawled. She suspected the next comment would include
the phrase, "a fine filly." She cut him off quickly. "Just the asparagus and directions."

"If you're sure," he responded, his eyes raking over her the
whole time he bagged up the stalks. "You just need to go up to
60th there and take a right. Go through downtown and when you
hit Timpson you take another right. You can't miss it. Just look for
the virgin in the bathtub."

Typical, she thought. The male species learns early. Then
they never miss an opportunity to leer and make suggestive comments. Even when they're old and demented—like her father. His
frontotemporal dementia was advancing predictably—the increasingly unwelcome comments toward her revolted Avy. She'd never
learned—and didn't want to know—how he had offended the
home care staff. The fall down the basement stairs may have been

only confusion in the middle of the night, but could also have been complicated by unsteadiness from the FTD.

It's a medical condition, she reminded herself again. He can't help it, but does that explain everything? His shocking words to the lawyer months back continued to drill into her skull in unguarded moments, like a woodpecker returning to a dead tree to dig for insects. Instead of removing them, though, the drumming just beetled his words deeper. He had always been able to hurt her. Why should it be different now? "As they live, they die," she had heard from a hospice nurse at the agency. He continued to be the "patient" she had the most trouble contending with.

Meanwhile, she flew down the sand and gravel road forgetting to watch for number 4776 or a bar sign—The Virgin in the Bathtub was it? I must have passed it, she thought, maybe the last corner where that run-down building looked deserted. She turned around in a driveway that warned, "KEEP OUT—STAY OUT," and drove slowly southward, checking mailboxes for the number.

Young leaves on mature hawthorns and pin oaks lent afternoon shade to the roadside. Their roots protruded from the steep sandy bank that formed a natural barrier on the left. Daylilies bobbed in patches of sunlight on the peaks of the right bank. The roller-coaster of a road was hillier than any she'd encountered since traveling these back roads for her job.

This work was a far cry from the hospital, but until she could figure out what to do with her father, she needed the flexibility it offered. He really wasn't safe to be alone unless she checked on him at least once during the day. And even then, she worried. She needed to finish up this day and make it home as soon as she could to prevent any further episodes like the one that had forced her to stay in the first place. Her father was getting around again in the house—unsteady but refusing to use the cane anymore. She worried he would overdo, or try to climb the stairs, or that he would leave the house, fall, and reinjure himself. The concussion had left him more addled than ever. But the remaining rib and sacral pain so far had seemed to keep him content to stay at home and muddle about with Alex.

While allowing the car to steer itself over the rutted road, she pulled her laptop from her bag to check the information. As she remembered, the address read 4776 Timpson.

"Spurge! Where is it?" She decided to try calling him again and hoped he would answer. "Maybe he never left the hospital," she muttered. "That would certainly make my day more manageable."

She popped the cell phone off her belt clip and punched in a few numbers. Nothing. The screen was lifeless. She flung the useless phone over her shoulder and it sailed out the open window.

"Bull thistle!" she cried. "Garlic mustard!" She had noticed these invasive plants overtaking the native ones as she skidded to a stop. She threw the car in reverse and backed up to the patch of garlic mustard. She got out of the car and tramped into the weeds, muttering their names again to express her frustration. The tangled thistles reached out bony fingers to grasp her skirt.

"Motherwort!" she yelled, although there was none to be seen. It was one of her mother's favorite expletives, and she felt better imagining them screaming it together and laughing. But the phone might have landed anywhere, and she had to find it. Her limited cash flow was needed for more important things than replacing a cell phone lost in a fit of pique.

Avy stepped into the sunlight bathing a gravel drive and felt the late afternoon breeze tickling her ankles. It had been a long time since they'd had sun like this. She looked back at her Focus, soundless in the shadow of a huge slippery elm dripping with Virginia creeper vines. A catbird mewed in the cottonwood thicket. "Okay,"

she told herself, "take it down a notch and come up with a system."
Beyond the driveway, the land fell away into a shade-dappled hollow. She noted pale pink spring beauties clustered among the roots
of an oak sapling. Cutleaved toothwort and daisy fleabane pushed
up from the ground on slim stems. A profusion of winter-killed
brush spoke of the variety of wildflowers that had died there while
she still enjoyed the lupines and forget-me-nots in the meadows
of the Rocky foothills. Avy filled her lungs with the mixed scent
of sun-warmed grass and leaf mold, then descended onto an overgrown pathway in the brushy hollow, avoiding stepping on the
early spring flowers. The path wound back and forth, as if children
had used the little glen for a game of follow-the-leader. Obediently,
she followed its labyrinthian path, and discovered her errant phone
lying at the base of a makeshift shrine, a bathtub upended in the
ground sheltering a statue of the Virgin Mary.

"The virgin in the bathtub." Avy shook her head, genuflected
to retrieve the phone, and turned to retrace her steps. That's when
she saw the mailbox, dragged aslant by the Virginia creeper vines
choking it. She pushed through the leaves and saw the numbers
4776 painted inexpertly on the side.

When she looked up the hill, she thought she could see a face
peering through a smeared picture window and a wisp of smoke
rising from the end of a lit cigarette. The figure retreated and she
turned back to her car.

Chapter 44

Her face reflected the late afternoon sun's glow as she climbed
from the driver's seat and swung the car door shut. She
couldn't repress a grin after finding her cell phone at the feet of
the Virgin. So, she could assume Mr. TenHaven was Catholic.
She added that to the few facts she had: Sixty-seven years old.
Widower. Son Arnie was closest relative. Fractured tib-fib from a
crushing accident while doing house repair. A concrete block fell
on his leg? Something like that. She noted the overturned wheelbarrow. Wooden 2x10s lay strewn a few feet from it. A car jack, of
all things, was wedged in the opening of the crawl space under the
house. And emphysema, she remembered, complicated with pneumonia after the surgery. By reflex, she took a deep breath to fill her
own lungs and inhaled the scent of honeysuckle and fresh-cut pine.
Someone had recently built the wheelchair ramp running up to the
deck. She could smell the newly hewn lumber. Professional job, she
thought, heading up the incline toward the screen door at the back
of the house. Sparrows burst noisily from a thicket of lopsided bird
feeders planted in a patch of grass as she rounded the corner to the
back door.

She balanced her bag on the railing and stood there, surveying the scene. "What a great view," she said, "except for the junk
piled against the side of the garage." Rotted lengths of lumber
were crammed tightly into a fifty-gallon burn barrel, all that was
preventing a pile of sagging plywood sheets from sliding to the
ground. A stack of five-gallon plastic buckets overflowed with a
paint-splotched drop cloth, a broken wooden handle, and half a
dozen stir sticks. Rolls of fiberglass insulation were soaked from the
recent spring rains. The rusty tongue of an old wooden trailer disappeared into the wild parsnip that softened the edges of the junk
pile. Beyond that, the side yard fell away to what could be a creek
bed, judging from the cattails and cottonwood saplings lining its
course. They were backed by more of what she had seen along the
road, ancient oaks and hawthorns. She thought she could pick out
a raspberry patch on the north side between the garage and the
creek. A couple of sparrows returned to a platform feeder, ignoring
her as they pulled seed from the base.

"Since you're here, you might as well come in, honey," a voice
called from inside the house. Embarrassed at being caught idling,
she wheeled from the railing and entered the house with a smile
plastered on her face. The door clattered shut behind her, startling a
skinny black cat. It flew off the kitchen table, sending the remains of
a TV dinner tray's crusted mashed potatoes skittering onto the floor.

"Great," Avy murmured, smile vanishing. "I haven't had
enough bad luck today? Now a black cat!" She picked up the foil
container and dropped it on top of the overflowing trash in the
wastebasket. She sighed deeply but immediately regretted it. Her
inhaled breath nudged the stink of rotting food up from the trash.
She pulled out her antiseptic hand cleanser from the pocket of her
lab coat, rubbed it into both hands, and held them up to her nose

for a moment to dispel the odor. Then she followed the tail of the cat and the sound of a rattling fan into the darkened living room.

She set her heavy bag on the scattered newspapers by Mr. Ten-Haven's well-worn La-Z-Boy and held out her hand. "I'm Aviana Lehrer, the nurse from Alliance Homecare."

He sat tipped back in the recliner with his feet dutifully propped up on the footrest. The wheelchair stood positioned on the right, between her patient and the oscillating fan. The cat jumped onto the arm of the chair.

"Bernie," he said, shaking her outstretched hand. "And this is Capone, my guard cat." He was a big man. Even in his current state she could see that. His legs protruded from a pair of blue and green plaid shorts, displaying prominent gnarled knees. His right lower leg, encased in a cast covered with signatures, extended well beyond the footrest. She puzzled over why a belt was looped around the ankle, but let it go. Sinewy chest muscles showed through his thin, ribbed undershirt. It was hard for her to tell if the barrel chest had developed from years of manual labor or from smoking. She ignored the wisp of smoke dancing in the fan's breeze for now. His grip on her hand was mercifully brief.

"Have a seat," he said, stretching to hook a wooden chair bottom with his thumb and last two fingers and drag it across the hardwood floor. His index and middle fingers were missing at the first knuckle on his left hand. The effort loosened a wave of perspiration odor and a fit of coughing. She guessed that they must have been too shorthanded in the hospital to give him a bath. He hacked something into a tissue and Avy knew she'd need to take a look at it. Later.

"Now tell me why everybody thinks I need a nurse."

"Well, let's talk about it and see if you do," Avy said.

"I like your thinking, young lady," Bernie said and grinned.

Avy risked this tentative beginning by asking first to use Bernie's phone. "I can't get any signal on mine, and I need to check in on an older gentleman a moment before we concentrate on you."

She was almost always able to get home by 4:00 so her father wouldn't be left alone in the early evening. Evenings were the worst. As the sun slipped into the west, his mind slipped away too. It would be nearly dark when she got home today. The phone went unanswered. Not surprising, but always a bit worrisome. She turned back resolutely to Bernie.

"Sit yourself down, then," he ordered. "I guess you want to survey the damage first. Damn fool thing of me to do. I should have waited for Arnie's help—Arnie's my son—but he's so busy I didn't want to bother him."

Avy tried to focus on her client, but her father's embittered face kept intruding on her thoughts. She wondered again why Jared hadn't noticed his father's decline before he left for college. Maybe he just chose to ignore it. Her father had taken early retirement to write—or maybe, she considered, he had been let go. But as far as Avy knew, he had never published anything. Her guardianship had finally come through, and she'd taken over from the guardian ad litem just this week. She'd made a follow-up appointment for her father with the neurologist Dr. Nanninga had recommended. She hoped she would soon have a better idea of how to care for him and what to expect in the future.

"If you want something done right, do it yourself," Bernie said, interrupting her thoughts. He'd always had a knack with things, he claimed. Could figure out how to do most anything he needed to, and could fix whatever needed fixing. "Fact is," he bragged, "I built this very house almost forty years ago. From foundation to chimney cap and everything in between and did just fine, thank you very much."

She suspected this was a well-rehearsed statement.

"Course you expect a few things to start going after that long," he admitted. "That's what got me in trouble, trying to shore up the flooring under the bathroom. Arnie told me, back when he helped me haul out the old tub, that the floor was rotting out, but I just put down some new plywood, hooked up a scratch-and-dent Sears special stall, and called it good. I was going to put down some linoleum, but when Rowena took sick it just didn't seem all that important. Arnie won't let me hear the end of it now."

"Rowena?" she asked.

His mouth hung open and his eyes glistened with sudden moisture. He sighed. "My wife died a year ago last winter."

"I'm so sorry."

He responded with a grunt through pursed lips and a quick nod in her direction before averting his eyes to squint through the picture window.

Avy waited for him to speak.

He sighed again and, still peering out the window, continued.

"I don't know how she managed to put up with me all these years. She had the patience of a saint. But when she got a plan in her head"—he smiled—"she found a way to make it happen, with or without my blessing."

He cocked his head toward the road down the hill outside the window, inviting Avy to picture it with him.

"Two summers ago, Rowena went and took a scythe down the hill and whacked through the brush all morning. She cleared a winding pathway and called it a labyrinth. Then she started in on me to help her build a shrine down there for her statue of the Virgin Mary. I'd been in the middle of another house renovation project and I'd just installed a brand-new shower in place of the original tub. It was long overdue since the plumbing had been leaking for who-knows-how-long and the floor had begun to sag from the rotting plywood of the sub-flooring. Rowena dropped one of her prescription capsules to show me that it rolled downhill toward the tub, so I couldn't put it off any longer." He grinned. "The old porcelain tub sat out behind the garage for months where my son, Arnie, and I had hauled it. So Rowena's inspiration involved me dragging it down the hill, digging a three-foot hole, and burying it with the curved end sticking out of the ground. She wanted to decorate it with a row of little blue tiles." His fingers mimed how she planned to arrange the tiles.

"When I asked her what the Virgin would think of spending all her days in the arch of an old bathtub, Rowena said that the Virgin was used to strange accommodations and that she would dignify the ordinary. 'Dignify the ordinary,' I thought. Whatever that meant. I put it off. All this veneration stuff she'd gotten into gave me the willies."

He shook his head. "When I finally understood how important it was to her, it was too late. She was sick. I hurried to construct it, according to her wishes, hoping that by honoring Jesus' mother, as Rowena did, maybe I would get the Virgin to put in a good word with her son about healing my wife.

"Rowena was never able to get down the hill from the house to visit the shrine. Instead, *I* visited the Virgin daily for months while Rowena's skin gradually lost its color till she, too, appeared to be made of porcelain. On the last day of December, I went down there, dropped down on the cold rock and stared at the silent statue. The outstretched arms offered nothing but two handfuls of cold, heavy snow. She died that night."

He stopped, breathing hard, his shoulders slumped in the chair.

"Mr. TenHaven, I—"

"Bernie," he insisted, turning back to smile at her. His shoulders straightened. "Anyway, last Friday I noticed some paint peeling off the side of the house by the foundation. The wood felt a little mushy, so I thought I'd better check it out. I got down on my belly to shine a light into the crawl space and I could see the joists were rotting out." Deep moist coughing interrupted him briefly. He cleared his throat and resumed. "So I picked up some 2x10s to reinforce 'em. I was loosening up the cinder blocks to get at the first joist when one of the damn things fell on my leg, and here we are."

She made a mental note to call Arnie to see if the house was up to code. It was way beyond the standard routine of checking for working smoke detectors, running water, and stair railings.

"My son Arnie," he said, as if he heard her thoughts, "is a building contractor and has a whole bunch of people working for him. If you can call it work," he said. "They seem to be sitting on their hands a lot from what I can see."

His medical history went quickly after that. There was nothing wrong with Bernie's memory as long as she could keep him on track. Her strategy was to swivel the laptop to face him. That way he could see how many questions she needed straight answers to. She was nearly finished when Arnie showed up at the door with three bags of groceries and Bernie's new medications.

With Arnie's insistence, Bernie agreed to an evaluation by Ryan, their no-nonsense physical therapist, but father and son both refused the support of an occupational therapist. Arnie showed her how his wife, Tracy, had moved everything in the kitchen and bathroom to where Bernie could reach what he needed. Just like Avy had done for Lydia and for her father. The cat trailed after her, growling a warning.

"Meddlers," Bernie muttered *sotto voce* from the living room. Tracy had also picked up a reacher, and Arnie had put up a grab bar next to the toilet. Avy was impressed.

"No need for all of that," Bernie yelled from the La-Z-Boy. "I could have hauled my ass off the toilet with the towel bar!"

Arnie grinned at her. "See what you're up against?"

"I specialize in obstinate." She cocked her left eyebrow, turned on her heel, and marched back into the living room.

In her own mind, Avy had established a rationale for nursing visits. Bernie's lung capacity was pretty limited and her stethoscope had picked up crackles in both lobes. The glob of phlegm she inspected in the tissue was grayish-green. Until he finished the course of antibiotics that Arnie had just delivered, she knew she should keep an eye on him. Especially if he was smoking on the sly. Later, they'd worry about what might be happening under the cast. But it was Bernie's decision that counted.

"Why don't we finish this up tomorrow, Bernie?" she said, after making sure he knew how to take the pills and use the inhaler. "What do you say? Can you stand seeing me again or are you going to sic Capone after me?" She scooped the cat up from the floor at her feet and faced Bernie. Capone pressed against her chest and purred.

"I can see how well that would work!"

"I'll come first thing in the morning," she promised.

"Not too early," he grinned, signing his permission. "I don't want you seeing me in my skivvies."

Chapter 45

Her workday had ended early for a change, and she felt rootless. She wasn't ready to return home, but she had nowhere to go. She realized that she was a mere half mile from where Andrew's mother, Lydia, lived. She hadn't seen her in over a month, but Monica had told her that she'd been discharged from Alliance a few weeks ago. It would be good to stop by and see how she was doing.

When she pulled into the driveway, she found Lydia sitting on the front porch, weaving a grapevine wreath. At her feet stood a basket of forsythia. As Avy stepped out of the car, Lydia's face lit up.

"What a treat to have you stop in! It's so good to see you!" Lydia set the grapevine aside and stood to wrap Avy in her arms as she arrived at the top of the steps. She felt the renewed strength in the woman's hug. She stepped back, still holding Lydia's arms in front of her, and looked her up and down. Her hair was now nearly an inch long, and she had wrapped a floral scarf around her head, since it was impossible to style. She was dressed in turquoise capris, a white sweater, and espadrilles.

"Wow! You look amazing! Do you feel as good as you look?"

"I'm back to my old self again," she said. "I have to thank you again for getting me set up with the home care people. I couldn't have managed without them. And now I hear that you're working there, too. Monica's a bit of a blabbermouth!"

"That's right. I just finished seeing a new client who lives not far from here. I thought it was time I checked up on you to make sure you were behaving yourself."

"Well, sit with me for a few minutes. Do you mind being outside? It's such a beautiful day." It was a perfect spring afternoon, warm with a cooling breeze that carried the scent of lilacs from the bush in the corner. Lydia indicated another chair at the far end of the porch and Avy dragged it over. She had just been feeling like such an outsider. She gladly plopped into the chair and impulsively reached for Lydia's hands.

"How's your father doing, Avy? Andrew told me you'd decided to stay in town to help him. You were always such a dutiful daughter, but I'm sorry that you had to leave that great job you had out east."

"Yes, that was really tough. I was devastated at the time, but now . . . I don't know. The work is so different than what I had planned on. I'm still getting used to all the paperwork, and some days are really frustrating, but—can I say that I'm having fun?"

"Can you?" Lydia reared back as if in shock. "You were always such a driven young woman, I was never sure you knew what fun was!"

"I know! I feel like I've become a different person. I still regret having to resign my position out in Albany, but I'm really enjoying the people I'm getting to know. Most of them anyway. Huh. . . . I never let myself get attached to anyone since Mom died. I think I missed out."

Lydia was quiet, just nodding and smiling winsomely. "But you let *us* in—Andrew and me."

"You were so easy, always at the ready with treats and hugs." Her voice came to a stop. She squeezed the hands she was still holding, raised them to her mouth and kissed them. "You were my salvation, and I just left without saying goodbye."

"You had your reasons, dear, I understand that now. But I'll admit we worried about you terribly, not knowing what had happened to you. Your father didn't seem to know either—or at least if he did, he didn't say."

"It was cruel of me. I didn't care if it hurt *him*, though I don't think it did. But I didn't mean to hurt anyone else. I did let him know after a while where I was and that I was okay, but I should have let you know, too. I'm so sorry."

"All is forgiven. You did finally contact Andrew, so we could rest easy after that, even though we missed you—Andrew especially."

She looked into Lydia's eyes and saw the truth of both the pain she had caused and the forgiveness she was granted. She had been selfish and unfair, but still loved by these two. She felt gratitude opening up her chest like an egg cracking open to release a tiny chick, weak and helpless.

Andrew's car pulled in and Lydia waved. "He said he was stopping at the Carrabba's downtown to get takeout. I'm sure there's enough if you could stay for dinner."

She had dropped Lydia's hands to wipe her eyes. Her heart was feeling too tender now to accept the offer.

"I wish I could, but I need to get home and make sure Dad will eat. He's become so disoriented." She turned to see Andrew loping from the car with two takeout bags. "Hi, Andrew. It's great to see you! I just stopped in to check on your Mom."

"You can't stay for dinner? I've got Italian. There's plenty."

"Thanks, but I need to get back to Dad."

"Well, another time then." He squeezed her in a one-armed hug, holding the food at arm's length.

"Great. Let's do that." She headed down the steps and turned to wave. Before tears slid from her eyes, she backed the car from the driveway and headed for home.

Chapter 46

The woman drifted like an apparition through the background, with thin hennaed hair, in a pale dress of '40s vintage. A lurid smear of bloodred lipstick oozed across her mouth and onto the pallid cheeks. She stared in Avy's direction but didn't speak.

"My older sister, Elinore," the professor explained. "She'll be back with tea now that she knows we have company." Dr. Bieger sat deep in the center of a sprung camelback sofa, in the only space not loaded with newspapers and pipe paraphernalia. He puffed around the stem of the richly burled briar pipe. Avy had not asked him to stop. She was learning to choose her battles in this delicate dance of home care nursing. So different from the ICU, where the patients surrendered all control, often even their consciousness, to a team of medical personnel and machines. The mantra of home care was, "You are a guest in their home. They are in control." Besides, she preferred the earthy smell of the pipe tobacco to the fusty odor of the house.

Each home had a personality that revealed that of its resident, she had discovered. Some places were a battlefield of conflicting tastes and styles, just as the residents fought each other's wishes and

needs. Some, like Mr. and Mrs. Cairn's home, reflected a benign
and bland compromise. Devorah Weismann's house, where her
mother Abigail was the permanent guest of honor, paid homage to
their Orthodox Jewish customs. A retired professor of linguistics,
Dr. Bieger lived in a tomb of a house that enshrined the love of his
life—words.

Books from estate sales and thrift shops lay stored in musty
boxes on the screen porch waiting to be sorted. Shelves lined every
wall of the living room. The dining room table and chairs supported the Roman Empire, while ancient Greece had conquered
the china cabinet. Avy had to move a stack of *US News & World
Report* magazines to the floor in order to sit on the edge of a peach-
and-champagne upholstered wingback.

Dr. Bieger mentioned offhandedly that he used to live in the
house next door with his family—a wife and six children. He
confessed he had bought this place, a ramshackle Victorian, just
to house his books. Eventually he moved in, too, escaping his
unhappy wife, who, within the month, committed suicide. The
investigators informed him they had found her body wedged completely inside the ancient gas stove. She probably had not intended
to start the fire that had burned down the house and taken the five
youngest children, they assured him.

"My sixteen-year-old daughter, who was at work that night,
chose to go live with Elinore, with or without my blessing," he
said. "I was relieved. Then Elinore showed up on my doorstep one
September afternoon four years later. My daughter dropped her off
for a visit and never came back. She ran off in Elinore's car, with
money from the surreptitious sale of her aunt's house.

"Elinore's an undemanding companion," he concluded as his
eightyish wraith of a sister glided in over the layers of ancient Persian rugs, balancing a tea tray. "Thank you, dear," he murmured,

patting her hand. She smiled at him, half-curtsied toward Avy's perch on the edge of the wingback, and drifted back in the direction of her bedroom.

"So," she said, stalling, "how's the diet going?" Her eyes never drifted from the tray with its steaming Minton teapot and cups. Beside them lay a paper plate of Saltine crackers draped with what she feared were anchovies. Their limp gray forms elicited the revolting taste of the oily salted fish in her mouth. Dr. Bieger was supposed to be avoiding salt and eating a carb-consistent diet for his diabetes.

"Life is too short to bother about diets," he responded. "Old men should be left alone to appreciate their food and their beer and whatever other vices they still have the strength to enjoy!" He waggled his pipestem at her and slipped an anchovy-draped cracker between his brown teeth. Even separated by the heavily laden table, she could smell his smoky-sour breath.

She poured tea into the two delicate cups. Tea leaves swirled in the amber liquid like the bits of information she wanted him to drink in. She wondered how she would ever get him to swallow the bitter instructions that might keep him alive. The tea leaves slowly settled to the bottom of the cups.

She slid up the sleeve of his fisherman-knit sweater and wrapped the obese-sized blood pressure cuff around his ample arm. It registered 196/88, dangerously high. His hands were puffy too, she observed, as the depression of her thumb on the back of his hand gradually filled in. The same for his calves and thighs. He was retaining fluid. Through her stethoscope, his lungs sounded like water burbling over the rocks in the Campau River. Oxygen level, according to her finger meter, was 86. Not great. He could use oxygen. "How has your blood sugar been?" she asked. "Are you checking it daily?"

"I'm feeling fine," he insisted. "I put no stock in quantitative data. I'm a historian, not some damned capitalistic economist!" He did look a bit like Karl Marx, she realized.

"In order for your doctor to know what he's doing he needs to be able to measure the effects of the insulin with those numbers," she explained. Frustration made her scold. "He sent me here to see if we can get a handle on your diabetes, your hypertension, and your congestive heart failure. He wasn't happy when he saw you in his office last week and the lab results showed that the medications are not keeping all those problems under control."

"If he wants to judge my health by numbers, he's a fool," the professor growled. "By the numbers, I should have died in '44." His voice steadied. "I give him the satisfaction of taking the medicine his science prescribes, but that doesn't mean I believe it improves the quality of my life, or prolongs it any either, for that matter." Smoke rose in stubborn puffs from between the yellow-stained halves of his mustache. "And why should I want to postpone the inevitable?"

It was a battle she needed to pick, she realized, but first she had to figure out how she could win it.

"Sure you don't want the last one?" He hesitated only a second before popping the last morsel in his mouth, licking the salt from his fingers, challenging her to scold. Over tea—his laced with milk and sugar, hers black—she cajoled him into letting her come twice a week to follow his progress. Meanwhile, she'd think about how she could persuade him to comply, at least in part, with the doctor's orders.

When the tea was cold and she had packed up her bag, he asked, "You wouldn't be related to Calvin Lehrer?"

"My father," she said. "Do you know him?"

"He was my student, and then we were colleagues long ago. I have his book."

She frowned. "I'm not sure we're talking about the same Calvin Lehrer. I don't think he ever published anything."

"Classical Language and Lit? Grand River State University?"

She nodded mutely and he continued. "Not surprised you didn't know about it. I believe he was a bit disillusioned about his thesis in the end. I headed his dissertation committee. Though he had at least one sympathetic member at GRSU, I thoroughly disagreed with him!" His pipestem emphasized his point. "We frequently sparred about his superstitious need to prove that the Hebrew and Greek scriptures were God-inspired." He chuckled. "But I do admit, it was brilliantly written, a faultless defense. It just wasn't true. In spite of that, I was the one who encouraged him to get it published."

Stunned, she said nothing. The old man confided, "I think I finally convinced him, by the way, of the error of his thesis, but he just wanted to get the PhD and be done with it!" He nodded in self-satisfaction. "If I can trust my memory, he was headed for the ministry, 'preaching the Word,' but he decided to use his PhD for something more worthy." The pipe waved dangerously again in the air between them. She would have worried that the ash escaping from it would start a fire in the sofa cushion if she hadn't been distracted by this new revelation. "I was happy to have him on board at the university. He ended up *teaching* the word, the pure language, instead of *preaching* all the theological claptrap." He swept his hands outward as if to embrace his own world of words. "Language itself forms meaning and offers pure truth. And the truth will set you free." He chuckled. "I believe that's in the Bible!"

From her mother's journal, Avy had learned that her father was conflicted about his plan to go into ministry. She tried to imagine him as a minister and conjured up the memory of a stern preacher from her childhood. She even remembered the verse he was using—"It is not good for man to be alone." He halted his sermon to scold eight-year-old Auralei right from the pulpit. She had been swinging her brand-new purse absent-mindedly by the strap. When it broke free and flew across the center aisle it caused several pairs of eyes to stray from his face. Her family had never returned. She could imagine her father as *that* kind of a preacher.

She realized that her patient had stopped talking and was smugly puffing away, reliving his victory over an impressionable graduate student.

"You said you had his book? I'd like to see it if you can find it."

"Of course! It's in the Comparative Religions section upstairs. I'll give you a copy. As head of his committee, I have several—they may even be autographed!" He initiated a rocking movement, each forward swing boosting him a little closer to the edge of the sagging sofa. In six repetitions he heaved himself upright, steadying his bulk with a burled walking stick that matched his pipe. She stood to follow.

She set her bag down on the stack of magazines, shook off the turmoil of these new revelations, and reoriented herself to the purpose for being in this man's home. She hoped he would agree to let her colleague Ryan, the physical therapist, come now that she had secured her own welcome. Following his unsteady traverse of the overlapping rugs, she realized that if he toppled she couldn't break his fall without injuring herself.

"I'll need to make a stop here," he confided, halting before an open doorway. "Balzac for the bathroom," he whispered conspiratorially. He belched fishy breath. "I have nearly all of his novels in French and English." Beyond the bathroom door, she saw mounds of leather-bound volumes. On the edge of the sink, with a strip of toilet paper marking his place, she spied *Les Chouans*. "It may be a few minutes," he admitted. "You may explore the French

Revolution in the kitchen while you wait, then we'll go upstairs to retrieve your father's treatise."

She stepped carefully over a wave in the undulating floor. He must have dozens of these rugs, she thought, layered haphazardly over each other. She shook her head over the impossibility of the standard safety instructions to remove loose throw rugs.

Something was stewing away on top of the old gas stove in a huge ceramic crock covered with a square block of warped half-inch plywood. When she heard the scrape of the bathroom door closing, she couldn't resist a peek in the crock. She eased up a corner of the plywood.

Abruptly, she let the wooden lid clatter back down on the crock. She stifled a scream with her free hand, as cockroaches burst over the side and jumped across the gas flame to safety.

Motherwort! Motherwort! Motherwort! her mind shrieked. The roaches had scuttled so quickly out of sight that she had no idea where they were. No clue where to step or what to touch. Or not. The kitchen filled with a yeasty smell, like feet that had worn hiking boots without a change of socks for a week. It was some sort of home brew stewing in the crock.

She yearned for the sterile predictability of a controlled ICU and backed out of the room to stand rigidly by the stairway that would lead her to her father's manuscript. She glanced back into the living room to make sure her bag still sat atop the magazine stack, zipped shut as she remembered.

The professor emerged from the bathroom. "Ah. You're ready to go up? Be careful on the stairs." Each step was bookended by a stack of musty volumes, leaving little space to walk. She followed his slow ascent to the next level.

"Here we are, Comparative Religions. Now—Williams, Smith, Sharpe, Packer, Novak—yes, Lehrer. Two copies. Have a look."

Opening one, she read the lengthy title—*Consistencies and Discrepancies in the Jewish and Christian Scriptures: A Linguistic Analysis of the Bible in the Original Languages of Hebrew, Greek, and Aramaic.* Her father's signature stood out in flowing script beneath his printed name.

"May I really keep this?"

"Who better than you?" he answered. "When I'm gone—" His arm swept across the shelves and a wistful cloud passed over his face.

Chapter 47

It had been three weeks since she'd first found Bernie after losing her phone at the feet of the virgin. Their visits had fallen into a companionable rhythm. The road to his home was familiar now, and she reveled in traversing the back roads from Agnes on the dairy farm, first thing in the morning, to Bernie's on Mondays. She never did catch him in his skivvies. Bernie's pneumonia was clearing up after a second round of antibiotics and despite the smoking, although he still complained that his "breath was coming in short pants." She didn't get the joke until Bernie waggled the hem of his Bermuda shorts at her.

By now she had discovered the reason for the worn belt looped around the cast. He was in the process of transferring from La-Z-Boy to wheelchair one day when she walked through the kitchen door. By hauling on the belt's end, he could easily lift the casted leg off the foot-rest of the recliner. She held her breath, poised to lunge forward, as he hovered unsteadily on his good leg before dropping into the shuddering wheelchair.

After two and a half weeks of working with the physical therapist, Bernie wanted to show off today. He waited in his wheelchair on the back porch for her to put the Focus into park. A late-model forest-green Camry that she hadn't seen before was parked in the grass beside the garage. The sunlight bounced off the metallic shine of the hood. She opened her mouth to ask about it, but Bernie didn't give her a chance.

"Wait right there," he called from the top of the ramp. He performed a three-sixty spin on the fresh wood of the platform, then flew to the bottom of the ramp on the two rear wheels.

"Don't tell Ryan!" he yelled as he whizzed past her. "He'd have my hide."

"I'd be more worried about the wheelchair rental company if I were you," she scolded. "And what if you tipped? I'm not sure even *your* thick skull could take that kind of a crack!"

Bernie waved off her objections. "This is what I wanted to show you anyway," he announced. He maneuvered the wheelchair, without the acrobatics, over the gravel to the base of the ramp. For the first time, Avy noticed the nylon rope attached beneath the seat. It ran up the ramp, over a rusted eight-inch flywheel attached to the railing's upright post, and back to the bottom of the railing.

He grasped the rope beneath the railing and began a swift hand-over-hand, chanting, "Improvise!"

Next grip—"Adapt!"

Then, "Overcome!"

"Improvise! Adapt! Overcome!" until he gained the deck.

She had heard that slogan somewhere, but couldn't place it. She wondered if it was something in the home care training videos that sank into her subconscious. It would fit, she thought. We have to improvise all the time. It went completely against all her previous nurse's training, but like Bernie and others, she was learning to make do with whatever was available.

And adapt. She hated it but she did it every day. She shuddered. But even more, her clients had to adapt to big changes in their lives. Sometimes it was temporary, she thought, like Bernie's broken leg, but more often it's something like his missing fingers that he has to adapt to forever.

We don't always overcome, though, she conceded. She wished it was that simple. She headed up the ramp.

"Where have I heard that slogan before?" she mused, joining him at the back door.

"Probably from Clint Eastwood in *Heartbreak Ridge*—unless you're a Marine."

"Were you a Marine?"

"Once a Marine, *always* a Marine! There's no such thing as an ex-Marine. But I served in Vietnam, if that's what you're asking." He held up his left hand with its missing fingers. "Left these behind in Khe Sanh."

"Oh, Bernie, no!"

His face broke into unrestrained laughter. "That one always gets me sympathy," he said. "But, to tell the truth, I lost them to a fierce table saw." He shrugged in half-hearted apology as she wrenched the back door open. A burst of bubbling jazz riffs tumbled out into the crisp air. It struck her as odd. Bernie didn't seem the type for jazz and she'd never before been greeted by any music at his home.

She held the door open for him and looked back at the pulley system as he bullied his way over the threshold. Ingenious, she thought, but certainly not safe. Not by home care regulations. It reminded her of the zip line her neighbors, nine-year-old twins Duane and Darren, had rigged up from their second-floor porch railing to a tree house in their backyard the summer she was eight.

A double dare had sent her flying through space until the line snapped and she fell on her tailbone, cracking it on the oak tree's snaking root. Not tattling had earned her a place in the boys' club until school started the next week. She wouldn't tattle on Bernie either. Let Ryan be the bad guy, she decided.

"Is someone else here?" she asked. "I noticed the car. And now the music." The lively syncopation filled the house, but there was also a living presence in the harmony, a whistled improvisation that surely was not part of the recording.

"Yeah. That Japanese piece of junk. Nobody wants American made anymore. It's going to ruin the economy."

"But I've heard Japanese cars are really well made."

"Don't believe it! Anyway, let me introduce you."

She followed Bernie down the hallway toward the far end of the house. She'd never been invited into this section before. The music gained in volume. They passed the bedroom on the right with its unmade bed against the far wall. Across the hall, thick plastic sheeting covered the open doorway of the bathroom.

A young man, his wild blond hair covered in plaster dust, grinned through his beard and the thick plastic. Bernie yelled above the music, "My stepson Nathan—helps Arnie out when he's got projects where the customers aren't too picky."

"You certainly qualify!" the young man called out.

Bernie dismissed the comment with a wave, as if brushing words out of the air. He turned from the hazy plastic sheeting and wheeled into the light streaming through an open door at the end of the hall. The door had been closed on her other visits, shrouding the hallway in darkness. Nathan turned back to his work and resumed his whistling.

He's improvising a tenor riff, she realized. Clever.

Her step lightened as she caught up to Bernie's silhouette at the doorway.

"Arnie and I added on this room after the wife passed," Bernie was saying. "I don't let just anybody in here." He winked at her and bumped over the uneven threshold into the room.

The late afternoon sun poured through the windows lining three walls of the workshop. House sparrows scattered from the feeders outside to perch in the venerable burr oak overhead. They scolded the intruders through the screen, unused to the disturbance. On the left stood low cabinets topped by a Bernie-adapted tool bench littered with chisels, hammers, and Band-Aid wrappers that spilled onto the floor. A vise at one end held a chunk of basswood. The smell of fresh-cut timber rose from a stack beside the bench. Her face lit up as she inhaled the scent; sawdust always brought back memories of her mother. Wood shavings, disturbed by their entrance, slithered like dry leaves across the pine floor. Bernie wheeled himself up to a low table with a single wooden chair against the far wall, bathed in sunlight. A half-mug of coffee squatted forgotten next to a pile of crumbs.

Avy watched Bernie rummage in a cardboard box under the table.

"This is for you," he said, turning. He held in his weathered hands a small wooden figure.

"I can't"—she began automatically.

"Take it," he insisted. "I made it special for you."

Oh, rules be damned, she thought, reaching out. She accepted its tender weight from his hands. It was a bird, exquisitely carved. Infinite patience must have been required to feather it so carefully. The bird's head cocked to one side in expectation or curiosity, and a wing lifted as if testing the breeze.

"It's a sparrow?" she asked.

"Yeah." He shrugged toward the window. "One of those little brown jobs."

"LBJs!" She laughed. Among bird-watchers and other nature lovers, sparrows were affectionately lumped together under that acronym. It took patience and insight to be able to discern one type from another. An act of love to name them individually. "Let me see what else you're working on." This creativity was a side of Bernie she hadn't imagined. She wondered what made him show it to her that day of all days.

Bernie had a shoebox full and more, including one on the table that was partially released from a chunk of wood. "I used to carve all kinds—cardinals, chickadees, bluebirds—and when I was finished, Rowena would paint them. They could have fooled their own mothers they were so realistic. I wish I had kept some, but they all went to gift shops and such, before I knew there wouldn't be any more." His sigh was as wistful as a mourning dove's cry. It, too, fit the new movement of the music down the hall. "But I'm no good with the painting," he went on quietly.

He pressed his left thumb beneath his nose, looked at the hand as if in surprise, then held it out toward Avy. "Probably would have lost another finger or two if I had picked up a knife then! I didn't have the steady hand or the clear eye a carver needs."

She stroked the carved bird in her hands.

"The spring after Rowena died, I didn't do much but sit out in that old chair, with my back to this ramshackle house she was willing to share with me. Facing her sacred garden, as she called it."

His shaky hand lifted to indicate the base of the hill, the pathway she had walked a few weeks ago to come upon the statue. Avy realized suddenly that she had trespassed carelessly on Rowena's sacred ground, maybe the first person to set foot there since she died. Bernie may have stopped talking briefly, but slowly she returned her attention to his story.

"After a while I turned to sparrows," he said. "They were all around me in the yard, and sitting there in the summer sun, I just started to carve again." He chuckled. "And Alicia," he said, "my two-year-old granddaughter with Down syndrome. There's not a lot she understands, but she just loves LBJs." He turned to face her. "So, like the old Marine I am, I adapted."

Chapter 48

"A re you there, God? It's me, Avy." She sat cross-legged on the sofa, listening. Nothing.

"What did I expect? Answers from heaven?"

She closed her father's manuscript on her lap. Professor Bieger was right. Not that she could judge if the work was brilliant. Theology, philosophy, classic languages—all over her head. But it was a different man who had written this work than the father she had known growing up. Bieger had broken through Calvin's confidence in his thesis and changed her father's whole belief system.

She wondered who she might have been if her father had kept his faith. Her childhood might have been very different. Resentment for the cynical old professor filled her. She could taste its bitterness like the leaves of the mustard garlic on her fingers after she weeded it out of the old perennial garden early that morning. She rose to go upstairs in search of her father.

The door of her bedroom, the room she had shared with Auralei as a child and had reclaimed when she resigned herself to moving back in with her father, was standing wide open. The old leather suitcase was open on the floor, her mother's journals scattered across the floor. Her father stood at her dresser, pawing through the disheveled contents of a drawer.

"What are you doing?" she blurted.

Startled, he nearly fell.

"I'm going home," he said. "My wife must be worried. I don't know what's taking the taxi so long. I'll miss my plane!" He gestured frantically at the suitcase on the floor. "I had my bag all packed before the lecture, but now someone's put these smelly old books and things in it."

"Your bag is all ready," she assured him, quickly entering into his distorted world to calm him. "It's waiting in the hall by the front door." Deception was second nature by now. Since his head injury, his mental confusion was nearly constant, and she had to figure out her role in whatever place and time her father occupied at any moment. Then improvise, adapt—would she ever overcome?

"This is Dr. Bieger's room," she continued, struggling to keep the anger out of her voice. "You know he's lost without his books. Your room is right across the hall. Why don't you relax and I'll check on the taxi. There's plenty of time." She took his arm and they moved in step through the doorway.

"Thank you, dear. I don't know what I was thinking. Absent-minded professor, you know."

"Not so absent-minded, sir. You always find your way back to stay with us when you're in town. We feel like you belong here, Professor Lehrer!"

"What was your name again, dear?" he asked as she settled him in at his desk.

"Aviana."

"I believe I knew an Aviana once. It's a pretty name."

She checked her wounded reaction. "Would you like room service tonight, professor? We have a wonderful homemade chicken soup and fresh whole-grain bread on the menu tonight."

He was now leafing through a *National Geographic* story on Palestine and didn't respond. She eased his door closed and reentered her own room. She retrieved the wooden sparrow he had knocked to the floor and let the dresser bear her weight while she studied her reflection in the mirror. She was exhausted from playing this game. How long could she keep this up?

Chapter 49

It was Avy's turn to cover the weekend again, so late on Friday afternoon she made her plan for the weekend and called her patients. It should be an easy couple of days—only Fred and Nick on Saturday and Nick again on Sunday. Since it was the weekend, she knew Nate would be around to stop the infusion anytime, so with his approval she bumped Nick's start time up to noon. Fred she could see around 10:30. And she could still meet Andrew for their planned afternoon hike in the state forest.

The plan started to unravel already at 6:15 on Friday night. It was Dr. Vydkowski himself, calling to see if the agency could admit a patient the next day. Still, she thought she could keep the date with Andrew. She caught herself. Date? Really? It's just a hike, she told herself. No need to make it weird.

"Her daughter-in-law left a message on my machine asking for advice on what sounds like a nasty pressure ulcer," he explained. "I'm just getting to the messages now. I haven't seen Mrs. Quinlan in several years. The family can never seem to get her in here. I doubt they're following through with her medications since I would have been called by the pharmacy after a year for refill requests, but here's what she should have been taking." Avy took down the information, the little he had. "Just do whatever you think best over the weekend—I'll cover the order—and call me on Monday." He agreed to call the family and let them know she'd be out in the morning.

At 8:00 Saturday morning, she pulled up to the once-white farmhouse. The back door stood open and she reeled from the thick odor seeping through the rusted screen. She hoped it wasn't coming from her new patient. A pale girl, maybe a teenager, shuffled from the blue glow of the living room to the door. She wore a holey oversized man's T-shirt. That appeared to be the extent of her dress.

"Yeah?"

"I'm Aviana, the nurse to see Helen Quinlan."

"Oh. Better come in, then. That's her."

Beyond the screen door, Avy could see through the filthy kitchen into a cluttered room. A dining table was shoved to one side, overflowing with dirty laundry. The backs of five chairs supported mismatched sheets, spread out like crooked tent panels.

She gathered there must be kids in the house.

She pulled the screen door loose from the doorjamb as the girl turned her back and disappeared into the blue glow. A ginger cat slipped from between two of the garbage bags wedged behind the door and leapt onto the table, knocking over a glass of milk in an effort to drink from it. The rumble of a larger beast shifting position under a bed on the opposite side of the dining room warned her to watch where she placed her feet.

Her shoes ground kibble into the sticky pine floorboards of the kitchen as she approached the figure in the bed. The acrid odor increased with each step. Her patient lay curled like a child on the bare mattress, her eyes squeezed shut as if she wished never to open them again. She wore a flimsy polyester nightgown, tangled in the wrinkles of a pile of old towels bunched under her hips. The gown looked as though it had once been a powdery blue, but now bore stains, in various shades of brown and yellow, that had wicked all the way to her armpits. No wonder the family wouldn't bring her to the doctor, she thought. She backed away to the edge of the room.

"Are you Mrs. Quinlan's granddaughter?" she asked, peering into the living room. She could just make out the girl, chomping on a Pop-Tart on the sagging sofa. The toddler on her lap craned his neck to stare at her. Avy blinked to adjust her focus in the darkened room on what she recognized as a portable commode with a bare-bottomed child balanced over it.

"Yeah. I'm Joyce," the girl said. Her eyes never strayed from the television.

"Is your mother or father around?"

"Ma's in bed. Sleeps days. Works nights at the Wolverine factory."

"Your father?"

"Fishing with Randy."

"Any chance they'll be back soon? I need to have someone sign the consent form, and he's the next of kin." Mrs. Quinlan had vascular dementia, dating from a stroke in 1997. That was when Dr. Vydkowski and the health care system had lost track of her.

"Can't say," Joyce said. "Prob'ly be gone for days."

"Okay," Avy said. "I could accept your mother's signature for now. Could you wake her?"

Joyce's head finally snapped around. "Not hardly!"

"Well, I need a family member's permission before I can do anything, since she can't speak for herself."

"Yeah, whatever." She waved a dismissal and turned back to the television.

Avy decided that would have to do. "I'll leave these papers, then, for your mother to sign when she gets up," she explained to the side of Joyce's slack face.

Wary of what might be under the bed, she approached again and crouched by Helen Quinlan's face. She touched the fragile hand gripping the yellowed lace of the nightgown. The woman's eyes flew open, startled by her touch.

"I'm Avy, a nurse here to make sure you get better. Do you want me to help you get cleaned up?" she asked. The woman's brow furrowed.

She chose to take that as a yes, since she refused to leave the woman as she was.

"Joyce," she called, "I'm going to need a basin of warm water, several clean towels, a fresh nightgown and some clean sheets."

Avy heard the girl's exasperated sigh, accompanied by the complaint of the sofa springs. Joyce dumped the whining child from her lap and grumbled, "Basin's in the sink."

Joyce's bare feet stomped past the kitchen door, farther into the darkness of the hallway. Avy damped down her own exasperation using her controlled breathing, and returned to the kitchen. She dumped the crusted dishes out and scrubbed the basin with globs of her hand sanitizer. There was no soap in sight.

Joyce returned with a jumble of linens and stopped at arm's length from Avy.

She wondered if the girl had pulled the sheets from somebody else's bed, but they beat anything else there. She glanced over the laundry pile on the table and the tent of soiled sheets that had been left, unwashed, to dry over the chair backs. They still reeked of urine and feces. But at least the towels looked washed. The gown was simply a worn and faded cotton housedress.

Joyce stepped back in disgust as Avy gently eased Helen onto her left side to remove the filthy nightgown. She left the soiled towels and gown under Helen's left hip to soak up the water from bathing.

"All day I got my hands in that crap with the kids and they expect me to clean up after her, too," Joyce grumbled.

"Doesn't look like you're living up to expectations," Avy said through clenched teeth.

"Huh! Like to see *you* do it!"

"Perfect! Watch, listen and learn, because you're going to have to take better care of your grandmother if you don't want Adult Protective Services walking in here!"

Joyce's retreat halted abruptly and she spun around to face Avy and the form on the mattress. She heard the girl mumble, "Bitch," under her breath.

The threat had gotten the girl's attention. Avy assumed they got government money through the MI Choice waiver program to take care of Mrs. Quinlan and muttered, "Wouldn't want to lose that!"

She drew on gloves, turning her back on Joyce.

She really hated to call APS even in a case as bad as this, but she knew she would if the girl didn't shape up.

She held her breath and carefully peeled back the stinking rag that served as a diaper. There it was, a gaping sore the size of a child's fist.

"Sweet *Lythrum salicaria*!"

"What the—" Joyce gagged, peering over her shoulder.

"Maggots!" Avy spit out.

"Omigod," the girl cried, lurching backward.

The bare-bottomed boy jumped onto the sofa, knocking his brother in the head with his knee. The toddler began howling in rage. His mother whipped around at the sound.

"Shut up that crying or I'll give you something to cry about!" she snapped, and lunged at him with her hand raised, open palm ready to come down on his pink skin. Overhead, bedsprings creaked. Heavy footsteps thudded across the ceiling.

"Oh, shit! Now I'm in for it!"

The younger child dropped off the sofa and tottered around the corner, now whimpering softly. His brother bypassed him at a run and both slid under the sheet tent in their mutual eagerness to avoid what was clumping down the stairs.

Avy ignored it all, concentrating on fiercely picking out all the maggots with gloved fingers and dropping them into an abandoned cereal bowl she'd found on the floor. The fly larva had done an expert job of cleaning the decaying tissue from the ulcer, but still. There were more sanitary ways of completing that.

"What the hell's going on? Can't I get some sleep in my own damn house?" A lumbering woman trailed behind the angry voice into the room. "Only one who works in this dump. Think I could have some peace and . . ." The tirade stopped abruptly as Avy straightened up from her task.

"Oh. You must be the nurse Dr. V. called about. Didn't think you'd come out on the weekend," the woman said, forcing her snarl into a grimace masquerading as a tight smile. Joyce began to back slowly out of the room.

"Get back in here you worthless slut," her mother growled.

She wheeled back on Avy and asked, "Well, what do you think? What are we supposed to do with that?"

"*That?* You see her as a 'that'?"

Helen lay rigid, eyes sealed tight with what little strength she had.

"This is what we're going to do," Avy said, her words punching from her mouth like balled fists. "Joyce is going to help me finish bathing *your mother-in-law*. I'm going to pack her wound with antiseptic gauze, now that the *maggots* have cleaned it out for me. *You're* going to sign those consent forms on the table. When I come back tomorrow, these sheets will all be washed. She will have clean ones on her bed and she will *not* be lying in her own filth. You are going to do *all* of that—or I'll be calling Adult Protective Services."

That afternoon, she channeled all her pent-up anger into her legs, stomping along the trail ahead of Andrew, impaling the earth with the hiking poles he'd loaned her.

"Avy," he called. "Slow down! What's going on?" She spun around to face him, breathing hard. He had stopped several yards behind her, poles held loosely at an angle, his head cocked to one side in puzzlement.

She realized she was sweating through her T-shirt and her face felt flushed. This was no way to release the stress she'd carried with her from the Quinlan house. She'd blown past the speed limit when she was back on the highway, trying to put the scene behind her, but it was plain that she was still in fury's control. She leaned on her poles, dropped her chin to her chest, and blew out a breath that rustled the leaves on the twig in front of her face.

"I'm sorry, Andrew," she said, seeing the hurt in his face. "It was a rough morning." She took a few steps toward him and he met her halfway. "I was called last night to admit a patient to our services this morning, and she was living in a horrible situation, one of the worst I've dealt with. It made me so angry that someone could be treated the way she was. I held it together while I was there, but it's still affecting me. I'm really sorry."

"I'm sorry you had to deal with that," he said, "but I'm glad it wasn't something *I* did to set you off."

"Thanks." She blew out another volume of trapped air, accompanied by tears spilling from her eyes. Andrew reached a hand for her shoulder. She didn't step away but let him enfold her in a one-armed hug.

"Do you want to tell me about it?" he asked tentatively. It was tempting to spill all the details of the disturbing encounter, but that went against the privacy rules of HIPAA, and her own strong code of ethics.

She wiped her tears on his shoulder, embarrassed at her loss of control, but remained in the comfort of his body. "Acting like a principled professional is exhausting!" A rumbling growl escaped into the quiet of the forest. She giggled and pulled back. "I haven't eaten anything since I left the house this morning. You don't happen to have any granola bars, do you?"

"I can do better than that," he said. "We're almost to a lookout tower up ahead. I think that might be a good place for a picnic." Grinning, they hiked on, side by side.

Chapter 50

On Sunday, she left the squalid Quinlan house for last. She anticipated a long hot shower when she got home. At 1:30, she headed for the run-down house out in the sticks north of town.

Half a dozen garbage bags leaned into each other outside the back door. A mangy spaniel she hadn't met yesterday squirmed out from under the steps. His slobbery yawn ended in a high-pitched yip, sounding more like a hiccup than anything she could imagine from such a large dog. In spite of herself, she grinned at the dog and patted his head tentatively. Probably yesterday's monster under the bed, she thought. Encouraged by the rare response, the dog commenced a slow scything of the Queen Anne's lace with his tail.

She knocked resolutely on the door and heard shuffling footsteps approach. Joyce's imposing mother, June, opened the screen door on squealing hinges and stood aside to let her in. She wore denim stretch pants and a pink sweatshirt that read, "It's good to be Queen," in holographic letters peeling away from the dingy fabric. Chipped red polish stained the toes poking from orange chenille scuffs.

"Well, we did what you said." The screen door crashed shut behind June's back. "Got her on the commode twice yesterday. She *still* soaked the bed this morning. That bandage you put on yesterday stunk something awful. I threw it out."

Helen was lying flat on her back on a bare mattress again except for a threadbare towel under her hips and a corduroy throw pillow under her head. With her chin tilted forward, her face disappeared inside the collar of a flannel shirt feathered with dryer lint. Wisps of downy gray hairs lifted feebly from her forehead with each exhalation, then drifted back before being puffed aloft again.

"I can't be running to the laundry-mat every time she messes the bed." June opened the door and heaved another bag on the pile. The door slammed, shimmying in the jamb. Avy noted the table was now emptied of laundry and the tent of filthy sheets was gone.

Seven garbage bags full of laundry. No wonder it smelled worse outside the house today, she thought. It seemed a little better inside, unless she was just getting used to it.

"Just because I didn't have to work last night doesn't mean I can do this all the time. I can't afford to lose my job." June lumbered to a kitchen chair that had been drawn into the room, aimed her buttocks, and dropped. "Joyce's gotta do it, if I have to smack her to get her off her fat, lazy ass." June's enormous thighs swallowed up the red plastic seat of the sturdy metal chair. Avy commanded her facial muscles not to draw her mouth into a sarcastic grin. She focused her attention on the frail body in the bed, gently positioning Helen on her side to examine the bedsore.

"Can't expect much from Roy even though it's *his* mother, not mine," June continued, rocking back and forth on her squeaky metal throne. "He's as useless as a bucket under a bull. And that idiot boyfriend of Joyce's is only good for making babies and swigging beer."

Helen must have been on her back for only a few minutes before she arrived, Avy surmised. There was only a little drainage on the shirt and the wound looked clean. She hoped maybe she wouldn't have to call APS after all. She'd take it one day at a time.

She hated alerting Adult Protective Services. The last time she called them to a situation like this, the entire family had disappeared before APS arrived. She never saw the poor man again.

With some basic teaching, daily wound care visits for a while—she ticked off in her head—a social worker and an aide, maybe she could make this work. She'd report in to Dr. Vydkowski tomorrow and hope he was okay with the plan.

"You've made a good start, June," she conceded. "Thank you. I'll need to start working with Joyce today if she's going to be the one doing most of the work after this. I've brought along some bed pads that should cut down on the laundry. Can we help you out, too, with a home health aide a few times a week to give her a thorough bath and shampoo? Then Joyce can just clean her up in between if she has an accident."

June stopped rocking.

"It's covered by her Medicaid benefit," Avy rushed to add. "It won't cost you anything." She went on, "I think a social worker might also help."

"No social worker," June snapped. "But the aide, yeah."

Okay, she thought. It's a start.

Chapter 51

By the first of June, Abigail Rosenberg could take a few steps with a walker. The *chasuna* was only a week away—next Tuesday evening—and Ryan was right. She'd come so far, but it was impossible that she would dance at the wedding. Abigail ignored their pessimism.

She showed off her new dress, a royal-blue brocade that set off her hennaed hair as Grace held it up against her tiny chest. A set of sapphire and silver earrings with matching choker and bracelet would transform her into the queen of Israel.

"*Sefirat Ha'Omer* is past! God be praised!" she cried. Weeks before, Abigail had explained *Sefirah* was a seven-week period of semimourning for orthodox Jews, its history buried in plagues and death. During *Sefirah*, no haircuts were allowed, no listening to instrumental music, no dancing, and no weddings. It began each year the day after Passover. This year it had also begun with Abigail's stroke. Her own body held the sign of semimourning, half of her weakened and anticipating the renewal promised after seven weeks.

"Time for celebration!" she cried. "As the Scripture says, 'There is a time to mourn and a time to dance.' Now is my time to dance!"

She continued, not allowing Avy to object: "The Scripture also says, 'Then maidens will dance and be glad, young men and old as well.'"

Avy considered pointing out that, though "the Scripture says" old men will dance, it doesn't say old women. Even if she felt like mentioning this, however, Abigail was too excited to quibble over gender issues.

She attempted to initiate the visit routine while Abigail launched into a description of the coming *chasuna* in great detail.

"Both the *kale* and the *khosen*—the bride and the groom—fast for the entire day to honor their new beginning together. They keep separate, the bride with her female relatives and friends and the groom with the men. There is much praying and well wishing. In the groom's quarters is held the *tanaaim*—the handkerchief ceremony where the groom takes a handkerchief from the rabbi to show his intention to fulfill his obligations in the marriage. Then finally he joins the bride for the *bedecken*—when he covers her head with the veil. All the while there is eating and drinking by the family and guests. Such food! Finally, the guests gather outdoors— because the marriage is to be under the stars as a reminder of God's promise to Abraham that his descendants would be as numerous as the stars."

Avy nodded appropriately, smiling while holding up the blood pressure cuff.

"All right! All right," Abigail agreed reluctantly. "I'll be quiet so you can check my blood pressure, but you will see it is fine."

Abigail was not satisfied until she had described the whole ceremony: the *chupa*, or wedding canopy under which the final ceremony would take place; the circling of the groom seven times by the bride and the mothers of the bride and groom to ensure his protection from evil; the reading of the *ketuba*—the contract that would legalize the marriage; the bride and groom both drinking from two cups of wine to show willingness to encounter both joy and sorrow together; the placing of the ring by the groom on the bride's finger to seal the agreement; and the groom crushing a wine glass underfoot to create noise and frighten away any evil spirits that wished to disrupt the couple's happiness.

Avy's head swam with images and she acknowledged a yearning she had long denied. There was no *chupa* in her future. No religious traditions. No loving family like Orli's to celebrate her.

And further, how was she supposed to grieve what she had lost? Her many losses of the past and now she was losing her father just as she had begun to understand him a little. She didn't understand the relationship they now had. What was she supposed to believe? Abigail's *Sefirah* was over, but Avy didn't even know where to start. No amount of spilled blood on a doorpost or noise from a broken glass had protected her *or* her mother. Evil had not passed over them. Since her mother died, Avy had lived a different kind of Passover. Passed over by her father. Passed over by her brother. Passed over by her sister. Passed over by the board of directors at Saint Stephen's. Passed over by every man who had ever shown even a glimmer of interest—except maybe Andrew. She felt that she'd lived through a hundred pass-overs and just as many semi-mournings with a little bit of herself dying each time. But she still hadn't reached the celebration.

Abigail's voice drew her back into the room. How much of the description Avy had missed, she had no idea. Automatically she had documented Abigail's vital signs, breath and heart sounds in the computer record. She was already at the mobility and self-care questions.

"And then the dancing!" Abigail exclaimed. "You've never seen such dancing!" And, of course, more food, more drink, and more dancing, she explained, as Avy assisted her to stand. She took two shuffling steps with her walker, laughing triumphantly. "I will dance at Orli's wedding!"

"From your mouth to God's ears."

"*Omeyn!*"

Chapter 52

This was Avy's first trip to the third floor, the attic that he used as his bedroom. "Hey," she said, stopping short behind Professor Bieger, who was wheezing on the second-floor landing. "Have you given any more thought to an aide to help you wash up?" The only working shower was on this level and, trailing behind him, she could smell that the climb was an effort.

Avy had released her resentment of the professor in the last few weeks. After all, her father had been an intelligent man, more capable than most of defending a position. His dissertation proved that. But apparently, he had failed to convince himself. Bieger had simply opened her father's mind to an alternative—logic. And reason was more compelling to him than mystery. She could understand that.

"No need. I'm fine just scrubbing down at the sink," he said, as she had expected. "Who needs a bath every day anyway? Hell, in Sagan we only got two cold showers a week!"

"Sagan?"

"Stalag Luft III. The POW camp. Now, I could tell you stories . . ." His voice trailed off as he climbed the last steps to the attic landing. "But that's another day." He took a deep breath, opened the door before them, and stepped into the lofty room. She was struck by heat, rolling over her like a wave. It was only June, but the attic room felt like August had set up housekeeping there. Moisture gathered in all her body's crevices.

They had reached the attic as the culmination of her tour of his singular library. It had begun weeks ago when she had first entered his home under orders to try to gain compliance with his diet and meds. She had made some progress with his medication use, as evidenced by the numbers he scoffed at. And she had been on the second floor that first day, to retrieve a copy of her father's dissertation in Bieger's Comparative Religions section.

On the way, he had proudly shown off each room, hall, staircase, and cubbyhole—every one stacked with books by category.

"I keep them separated so they don't fight," he explained, indicating the shelves lining each side of the attic room. Dust rose from under his paternal pat on the spine of *The Russian Revolution* on the Soviet history shelf. Czarist History lined the wall across the wide room. Between the opposing ranks, in the center of the attic, stood a king-size bed hung about with mosquito netting gathered high in the rafters on an iron hook. From the hook, an electric cord dropped within the netting, ending with a naked light bulb and a frayed string cord.

"Not for mosquitoes," he said, chuckling, while following her gaze.

"Then why?"

"Bats."

Her nostrils flared and her shoulders hunched involuntarily as she scanned the shadowy peak of the twelve-foot-high ceiling. Among the cobwebs she sensed malevolent forms clinging to the rafters.

"They strafe the light at night while I'm trying to read," he said, puffing on his briar pipe. "They're a nuisance. Especially if they're on a suicide mission."

Dr. Bieger had unusual methods for dealing with nuisances. Like buying a spare house to hold his books, then moving in to distance himself from a disturbed wife. The charred stone foundation next door where his family had died was visible from the attic window.

The old professor pointed her toward a makeshift closet in an alcove under the northern eave. Against the wall stood a cabinet with at least a dozen six-inch square compartments; a pair of worn black dress shoes, badly needing a coat of polish, nested in each one.

She wondered why on earth he had all these shoes. Did he have a shoe fetish? But then wouldn't he be collecting women's shoes? And a variety? Whatever, she concluded, she was glad to be wearing tan shoes that day.

In stark contrast, above the black shoe collection, an eight-foot wooden dowel hanging from the sloping ceiling held dozens of king-size shirts in varying degrees of white. On a nail in the far wall hung a single black suit identical to the one he wore.

"Dr. Bieger," she began. "Why—" She waved her hand to encompass the odd collection.

"You never know when you'll need an extra pair of shoes," he said defensively. "Or a clean white shirt. I pick up spares when I see them at Goodwill."

Chapter 53

On her way down the rutted dirt road, she bumped past two ambulances and three patrol cars racing in the opposite direction. Her head snapped back to verify that it was Andrew driving in the third cruiser. The Focus was too low to the ground to risk increasing its speed, but her heart sped up as she maneuvered her way over the last three miles before turning into the familiar driveway. A mud-spattered brown pickup, its tailgate lowered, squatted in the depression in front of the garage. As she opened her car door, the grasshoppers took over the buzz in her ears as the air-conditioning ticked to a stop. A haze of dust settled on the metallic-blue finish of the car and clung to the dampness at her temples.

Joyce, face flushed, opened the screen door, a child on each hip.

"You just missed all the excitement," she announced.

"What's happened to Helen?"

"You saw the ambulances? Well, Grandma was in the one. She's okay. They're taking her to the old folks' home in the city. Just as well, I guess. Daddy was in the other one. He's not okay. Momma and Randy got put in separate cop cars."

"I saw the squad cars."

"Yeah, I told the dispatcher they might need some backup."
She grinned.

"Okay. You'd better start from the beginning. Is it alright to
go inside?"

The spaniel crept out from under the porch steps and slipped
in beside her, knocking her into the doorframe. Joyce dropped the
boys onto the sofa and turned on the TV, tuned to the Shopping
Network. She picked up the commode that lay in front of the TV
and carried it back to the dining room. Avy stared at the empty
bed. A soft depression in the clean sheets showed where Helen had
recently lain.

"Well," Joyce began, as Avy sank into a dining room chair.
"Daddy and Randy came home around 11:00 this morning. They
had a whole mess of fish in the cooler. Apparently, they kept drinking up the beer in it to make room for more fish, 'cause they were
roaring drunk when they got home."

Avy had been fortunate enough in the past days to visit the
house when the men were still gone.

"Momma was asleep as usual after working at the plant all
night, but Daddy yelled for her to get down here and clean the
fish. I tried to tell him I'd do it, not to wake Momma. You know
what she's like."

Avy had also carefully timed her visits since the first two days
to avoid the "Queen."

"He just shoved me out of the way and went on yelling for
Momma. I called for Randy to shush him, but Randy had already
passed out on the sofa—just dumped the boys on the floor.

"When I heard Momma coming, I grabbed the boys and
ducked in here." Both of the women's heads swiveled simultaneously to stare at the empty bed and Joyce's narrative stopped. Her
eyes glistened.

"What happened then?" Avy prodded.

Joyce had lost her train of thought. Her voice was filled with something bittersweet when she resumed.

"You know that yesterday she called me by my name? While I was bathing her? She knew who I was. And that got me remembering what it used to be like. We would sit right here at this table when I was in school, and she'd help me with my algebra homework. I forgot that she used to be really good at math. Huh." Joyce shook her head. "But then I met Randy and dropped out because of the baby, and Grandma just kind of drew inside herself, I guess. I wasn't really paying attention."

"Joyce, you did a really good job here learning to take care of her. I'm proud of you. What's going to happen now? What happened to the rest of your family?"

"Oh." Joyce's eyes cleared to a fierce blue. "Well, Daddy had come in, dragging all his tackle, and he happened to have the fillet knife in his hand—I suppose to make it clear what he wanted Momma to do. When Momma came downstairs, mad as a hornet, first thing she saw was Daddy standing there, blind drunk with a knife in his hand. I knew we were in for trouble, so I dropped the boys on the bed with Grandma and turned this here table on its side to keep them all out of the action." She paused. "I guess the paramedics must have put it back upright when they put Grandma on the stretcher."

"What happened when your mother saw your father with the knife?"

"Went for the knife, of course. Just like I expected. Wasn't hard to get it away from somebody as plastered as Daddy was, but still they both got cut up some, Daddy more than Momma. A fillet knife is really wicked. He was headed for her again when I bashed him over the head with the commode. Wish it had been full." Her face wore a lopsided grin—the first time Avy'd seen her smile. "He dropped like a day-old carp. Momma was bleeding pretty bad, though, so she grabbed one of Will's diapers and wrapped it around her wrist."

Joyce paused. In the background, the host of the Shopping Network was hawking a set of Wolfgang Puck cookware.

"Momma went back in the living room and kicked Daddy—I guess to see if I'd knocked him out good. Then she picked up the knife from the floor and raised it over him. I swear, Avy, she was going to stab him. I didn't hardly see what happened, but right then Randy grunted and rolled off the couch. He knocked her right off her feet. She came down on Daddy and the knife went right into his back. That's when I called 911."

A low keening sound began and Avy glanced back at the TV before recognizing Joyce as the source. As it grew louder, she wound her arms around the girl.

"What am I gonna do, now? I can't stay here. Once they're patched up they'll be back here and it'll be hell to pay. What if one of 'em ends up in jail? Avy, Momma knows I saw her stab Daddy. And much as I despise them all, Randy included, they're all I've got now Grandma's gone."

"And the boys?"

"Oh, God." Joyce pulled out of Avy's arms. "You see what a great mother I am? I don't deserve to have kids. They'll turn out as bad, or worse, as their father. I should leave 'em on a church doorstep." She picked up the toddler from the couch, bouncing him instinctively on her hip. His startled eyes searched Joyce's face.

"Can you help me find a place to put 'em? I heard of kids being left at fire stations. Then I could take off and manage on my own, I guess."

"Joyce! What are you talking about? If you try to give them up, they'll end up with Child Protective Services and be in foster care for ages. Anyway, fire stations only take newborns. Your boys are too old."

This is so out of my wheelhouse, she thought. Not to mention against any sort of regulation for my practice. But what will happen to these kids if I walk away?

"Okay. Let's think about this," Avy continued. "We agree that it would be a good idea for you to get away from this house, at least for now." Suddenly she thought of Claire, and the shelter at the church. Would they take Joyce and her boys?

"I can call someone who knows about this kind of stuff. She might be able to help you find a shelter for yourself and the kids."

"But I don't have any money! That's why I've stayed here so long."

"I don't think you'll need to pay. At least not right away. Let's just get you out of here. Why don't you get some things together for you and the boys and I'll make the call."

All the brashness had gone out of the young woman. Joyce made her way into the dark hallway, where Avy assumed she had a room with her boys. She found Claire's card in her wallet and dialed the number of the church.

Chapter 54

Avy arrived at Abigail's home early on the Tuesday of the wedding. The cloudless sky promised a starry canopy for that night's ceremony. Anticipating the joyful flurry of activity inside the house, Avy fairly skipped to the door.

But dismay, in the wide-eyed form of Devorah, greeted her inside.

"What's wrong, Devorah? Is it Abigail?"

"No, she's upset, but she's fine. It's Grace. She was hospitalized during the night with a gall bladder attack. She's recovering well after the surgery, but she'll be in the hospital until tomorrow at least."

"Oh no! You must be frantic without her help, today of all days."

"God be praised, I have enough help for the routine tasks, but I don't know what we'll do with Mama tonight. Grace was supposed to accompany her to the wedding. She's so good with Mother since your therapist showed her how to move her safely. No one else but Orli knows what to do, but obviously that's not going to work. Shaylah, Orli's sister, has little Bina to look after. And the rest of us will all be participating in the different ceremonies. I'm at a loss for how to manage her."

During this monologue, Devorah had been towing her by the hand to the apartment where Abigail held court. She stopped just outside the door to release her, touch the mezuzah, and kiss her own fingers. Then Devorah set her shoulders, breathing deeply.

Avy realized that Abigail would be crushed to be left behind; she'd been looking forward to it for months! She might not be able to dance, but she should be there to enjoy the celebration she had counted on. Avy feared what this would do to Abigail.

Devorah knocked lightly and opened the door, motioning Avy to enter. Abigail sat disheveled in her bed, still in her nightgown. Avy had expected weeping and agitation, but Abigail leaned calmly back on her satin pillows. The innocence of her elfin smile belied the wily gleam in her eyes.

"So, you would like to attend a Jewish wedding, no?"

"No! I mean yes, of course I would! But I can't! It's tonight—I have to work till late this afternoon."

"The ceremonies don't begin until 6:00," she argued. "You can meet us there. Devorah will be satisfied that I'm in good hands."

Devorah, pausing inside the door of Abigail's apartment, overheard.

"Mama, you mustn't ask such a favor of Avy. It's too much." She waved a hand in admonishment, warning her mother with an upraised eyebrow. "There's nothing more to be said about it."

"No, wait," Avy said. "I would be honored to assist Abigail tonight. After all she's told me about the wedding, I'd love to see it for myself." Her mind whirred. "I can make it work," she announced, "and I can try to get one of our aides here this afternoon to help you get ready."

She had agreed to Abigail's request on impulse, before considering all the ramifications. She hoped that no crises would occur and that she would have enough time to shower and change before joining them at the country club. She feared that she didn't have anything appropriate to wear until she remembered the blue silk hanging in the back of her closet, never worn. Her mind churned. Were the sleeves long enough? she wondered. And what would she do about her father?

The issue of her father's need for supervision was solved unconventionally. After seeing Professor Bieger that afternoon, she took him home with her, and the two men assumed their old battle positions over her father's ancient Scrabble board. She didn't want to think about the ethical ramifications of using one of her clients to babysit her father.

At 6:00 that evening, Avy watched the wedding valet drive off in her shining Focus, fresh from the car wash. She firmly banished any embarrassment that it was out of place among the Mercedes and Lincolns.

She inhaled to tuck in her abs, turned, and ascended the wide marble steps to the entrance. She found Abigail in the immense sun porch, chattering excitedly with the flock of women gathered around the bride. Orli was radiant in an embroidered lace gown, with a multilayered tulle skirt. She alternately whispered with her sister, hugged her friends, and listened attentively to the serious counsel shared by Devorah and the older women in attendance.

As Avy approached Abigail's side, the lovely old woman reached for her hands and pulled her down to sit beside her on the sofa.

"Thank you," she murmured. "May the Lord's blessing be on your head for giving this old bubbe her wish."

She wondered if the prickling on the crown of her head was the Lord's blessing. She didn't know what it should feel like.

Abigail held tightly to her hands and shook them for emphasis. "King David said to the Lord, 'You have turned my wailing into dancing,' but it applies to you as well."

Abigail's eyes were drawn back to Orli, as if the girl's heart was a magnet for her grandmother's gaze. Her face glowed with an inner joy. "Isn't she beautiful, my *shayna maydel?*" she exclaimed proudly to the women surrounding the bride. "As beautiful as the seven worlds. 'She will be a wife of noble character,' as the Scripture says. 'Her children shall arise and call her blessed, and her husband will praise her.'" The women nodded and, in unison, cried "*Omeyn.*"

As she gazed at Orli, Avy sensed that *this* prophecy, at least, would come to pass. She was so young, but already she showed wisdom, strength of purpose, and a firm devotion to her God. Not unlike her grandmother.

Suddenly, young men, all dressed in black suits and fedoras, burst into the room, chanting and clapping in rhythm as they led Benjamin, the groom, flanked by both his father and Orli's, into the crowd of women. In the center of the throng, Benjamin drew Orli's veil over her face. His father began speaking in Hebrew.

Abigail whispered in her ear. "He's asking the Lord to bless her with a home of Torah values, and with myriads of children." She continued to interpret for Avy each activity of the evening. The proud bubbe's excitement grew as the evening progressed.

For two hours, as they waited for twilight, efficient servers circled the guests with hors d'oeuvres: miniature spinach quiches, lamb chops, trimmed to bite-size and nestled in sweet potato mash, and best of all, dark chocolate lace candies.

"You certainly didn't exaggerate about the food!" she said.

"Or the wine!" Abigail raised a glass to ring against hers. She ate with relish and insisted that Avy try every new delicacy.

As she guided Abigail's chair through the guests in her rippling silk dress, she envisioned herself as a liveried driver of a horse-drawn chariot. Her passenger held court as if from a carriage instead of a wheelchair.

"Fayga! Herschel!" Abigail called out, waving to an elderly couple sipping wine on the terrace. Avy eased the chair over the threshold of one of a half dozen sets of French doors overlooking the terrace, trying to minimize the bumps to Abigail's tush caused by the uneven flagstones.

"Abigail! What a glorious evening for your granddaughter's *chasuna*. May you be blessed among women," Fayga cried.

"May God be praised, you are here to see it," Herschel said. "After what you have suffered."

"You shouldn't know from sickness, but if—God forbid—it happens, you should have this angel, Aviana, for your nurse and her tyrannical team of therapists to get you back on your feet." She laughed.

"Aviana," Herschel said. "You are from our *yeshiva*, no?"

"No," Abigail cut in. "She's a good Christian girl who is making your old sister very happy! Avy, this is Herschel, my brother, and his wife, Fayga." Gallantly, Herschel bowed deeply as Fayga elbowed him.

She wondered if she was the only *goy* in attendance and hoped she wouldn't commit any horrible faux pas. She wished she'd had time to do her homework on the proper protocol for gentiles at orthodox Jewish weddings.

Finally, she found herself near the front of a wave of exuberant guests. The wedding ceremony itself was about to start. They surged from the terrace down the hill, where the wave broke into two—one half, black-suited men, and the other half, women in all the colors of spring. She assisted Abigail to sit in a place of honor at the front of the women's side on the left. Abigail drew her down into the seat beside her.

"The ceremony is held under the stars, to remind the couple of the Lord's promise to multiply their children like the stars of the sky," she again explained.

"The promise of Abraham?"

Abigail smiled. "You remembered!"

She barely recognized the *chupa*. This dreamlike structure bore only a slight resemblance to the simple marriage canopy in *Fiddler on the Roof*. Its four pillars were festooned with hundreds of perfect roses—peach, lavender, and white—intertwined with white satin ribbons securing the corners of the silk canopy.

Abigail whispered commentary as Orli, Devorah, and Benjamin's mother circled the groom "seven times, a holy number, to protect the bridegroom from evil."

She had only scattered memories of Abigail's explanation of a Jewish wedding from weeks before, so the diminutive lady's whispered interpretation helped her to understand the Hebrew blessings, the wine sipping, and why the ring was placed on the bride's right forefinger. Yet even though she cried, "Mazel tov!" with the others when the groom smashed the wine glass underfoot, she knew she was still an observer, not a true participant in this community linked by a common history, faith, and tradition. She might enjoy, but she would never belong.

Overhead, star after star appeared as she wheeled Abigail over the flagstone walkway and through the French doors into the ballroom. Already a group of young men danced frenetically in a circle, sidelocks and fringes flying. The band wasn't the kind of wedding band she was used to. Tuxedoed musicians pulled traditional Jewish folk music from violins, saxophones, clarinets, and drums. Despite Abigail's previous descriptions, Avy was unprepared for the wild enthusiasm of the dancers.

"The women will dance over there," her charge said, pointing to a row of room dividers draped with white silk and ribbons that separated the women's area from the men's. Abigail greeted friends excitedly as they circumnavigated the crowded room.

She raised her hand to slow Avy. "I'm parched. Let's have something to drink first and maybe some fruit to give us energy for dancing," she suggested. "The women won't begin dancing quite yet."

Avy saw the buffet tables laden with fruit and more hors d'oeuvres. And dinner hadn't yet been served! She realized that if she didn't pace herself, the seams of her dress might give way.

One side of the ballroom held dozens of round tables with elaborate centerpieces featuring the same perfect roses that had been used on the *chupa* pillars. Beside goblets of chilled fruit were more tantalizing chocolates. She helped Abigail into a chair at one of the family tables, beside Orli's sister, Shaylah, and her six-year-old daughter, Bina, and sipped ice water. She, too, was thirsty. Abigail speared a red grape and chortled as Bina danced about, trying to catch the bubbles blown by her mother.

"You see how even the children dance for joy," she said, watching her great-granddaughter's effortless movement. Then she turned unexpectedly to face Avy squarely.

"You *must* begin to dance, Aviana," she urged.

"It's too late for me," Avy said.

Abigail pressed her lips together and peered into Avy's eyes. She spoke urgently.

"My heart is dancing tonight," she said, "but I know what you have tried to tell me all along is true. My feet will not dance.

They may never dance again. You must take my place tonight, yes? Please. Perform this *mitzvah* for me. God will bless us both."

There were no tears in her pleading eyes, though there were in Avy's. The guests milling about them blended into a floating mist of colors. The cacophony of voices and music melded into a rushing wind that threatened to break through her defenses.

"Abigail," she said after a moment, "you've shared with me all your counsel about dancing, from the scriptures to W. H. Auden. Now I have a word for you from one of my old favorites—T. S. Eliot." She dabbed at her tears carefully. "Now he *was* a good Christian," she teased. "He said, 'Except for the point, the still point, there would be no dance, and there is only the dance.' I doubt that this is what he meant, but if you will promise to sit *still* tonight, I will try to dance."

Shaylah had overheard. Smiling, she said, "Then it's time. The women are leading Orli to the dance floor! Come on. Bina and I will help you." She hurriedly transferred Abigail back into her wheelchair. Then Shaylah pushed her grandmother's chair around the partition so she could watch, as Bina pulled Avy along.

They grasped her hands and joined with the others to circle the bride. With their support, she found her feet shifting, skipping, and dancing a grapevine around Orli. Their triplet would break from the greater vine to join hands with others in small groups, only to return, grafting into the greater vine that now swirled like a maelstrom, eyes wild with delight. Devorah and Orli lifted their voluminous skirts and danced what looked, to her untrained eye, like a polka while the women clapped, stamped, and sang: "*Mazel tov and siman tov and mazel tov and siman tov!*"

Faster and faster, the rhythm leapt from the pounding feet into her chest as she was enveloped in the ecstasy of the dance. Then, in the center, the younger women lifted Orli on a chair and whirled her above their shoulders. Her carefully coifed hair loosened and danced about her radiant face, which glistened with perspiration. When the dancers brought her back down to earth, Devorah caught Orli's hand and together they led the group, laughing, on a wild serpentine around the room, till she realized they had circled Abigail's wheelchair. The old woman beamed, tears streaming down her face, the still point in the center of the dance.

Chapter 55

She had finally gotten an appointment with Dr. Nanninga on a Thursday about the persistent pain in her back. She couldn't ignore it any longer. He'd done a full physical with blood work, an X-ray of her back, and an MRI. On the following Monday he called her in for a follow-up.

"Well, I believe I have a clear picture of what's causing your pain." He clicked on the light box on the wall and slapped a film against it. Avy recognized the cross section of a vertebra and adjacent lung tissue. "Here's the culprit." He pointed to the image on the screen, sweeping his finger around an egg-shaped blob nestled between her right lung and the edge of the vertebra. "This is a posterior mediastinal tumor." At the words, she felt the room shrinking.

"It's most likely benign," Dr. Nanninga rushed to say, in a manner meant to be encouraging. "The margins are well differentiated and it doesn't appear to have invaded any adjacent tissues, but as you can see"—his finger paused at points around the blob on the screen—"it's pressing against your lung, spine, esophagus, and a number of nerves and blood vessels. Thus the pain you've been experiencing—and perhaps some other internal issues? Have you noticed any other symptoms beside your back pain?"

Avy wrested her focus from the pale egg shape nested where it shouldn't be—a tumor inside of her—to consider the question. The pain had become nearly constant, so any other issues seemed inconsequential. "I don't know if it has anything to do with this," she finally responded. "There always seems to be a logical reason for it, but my stomach has been acting up lately. I've vomited more frequently than seems normal, but it seems to happen with noxious smells or emotional upsets, and once when I had a head injury. Could that be related to this?"

"That seems possible. The tumor isn't impinging on your stomach, per se, but it may very well be irritating your esophagus, which may then produce a gag reflex. Anything else?"

"Well, my voice seems to give out quickly when I'm talking for a long time—which happens when I need to explain how home care works to a new patient."

"At this stage, it's hard to know if those things are related, but we should get that tumor out, since it's causing you such pain. I'll have my nurse call the surgeon's office to schedule you as soon as we can get you in."

As soon as they could get her in? Emergency surgery was never a good sign, she knew. Then why would he say it's probably benign if he's in a hurry to get it out? She mentally sparred with his words and their implications as she went about her day. In that specific area where the spine, the scapulae, and ribs formed a protective triangle, so much could go wrong. Lung, heart, spinal cord, nerve tissue, liver. It must be malignant, she reasoned. Her mother had died from cancer, she worried, and maybe she had inherited a gene that had developed into cancer, too. It could have metastasized from somewhere else in her body. Even worse, it could have metastasized *to* somewhere else—like her brain. Or her stomach? That would explain a great deal, she decided.

Avy had never thought of cancer as an invasive species, but now the word echoed in her brain until it topped her list of expletives.

"Cancer!"

Chapter 56

A ll day she had triaged the concerns of her patients above her own, delegating her own fears to lowest priority. But there was one more concern she had to address before she could allow herself to fall apart. Nick's condition when she had seen him earlier nagged at her the rest of the day. She'd found him flushed and wheezing, and even a bit disoriented. Though he had finished the IV regimen for the histoplasmosis earlier in the week and had been feeling well, these symptoms were new and troublesome. The doctor had ordered both a blood and sputum sample, which she had delivered to the lab that morning, on her way to her appointment with Dr. Nanninga. Now she hoped to put that worry to rest in a quick stop and let her mind wind down. She headed back out into the growing dusk.

In the mental whirlwind she'd been trying to control following her doctor's appointment that morning, she couldn't pay attention to anything outside the parameters of her immediate patients' needs, so nothing about the scene before her now struck her as odd: the front door open, the porch light on, the lights illuminating the shrubbery from every window in the house, the figure on the second-floor pacing across her view with a cell phone pressed to his cheek. She walked up the steps and into the house and the whirlwind struck her full force.

Tilda's hands fluttered toward her as she entered. "Something's wrong with Nicholas!" she cried as a burly sixtyish woman—her daughter, Jessie?—pushed the old woman aside to block Avy's path. But Avy veered out of the woman's reach and bolted up the stairs. The oak door at the top burst open and plaster dust exploded where it struck the wall, freckling her face as she balanced on the top stair.

"Who are *you*? Where's the *ambulance*?" the young man fairly screamed. Blue eyes bloodshot and terrified, he braced himself in the doorway. One hand clutched his trim beard and Avy thought he might tear it out in frustration. She heard strangled sounds coming from behind him and realized Nick was in serious trouble.

"Aviana, Nick's nurse," she explained. "You're Nate? You called the ambulance?"

He nodded, long blond ponytail brushing his shoulders as she ducked under his arm. Something else registered in his eyes—surprise—as she flew into the bedroom.

Nick lay collapsed in a nest of pillows, gaunt and exhausted from coughing and the effort to breathe, shivering under a comforter. Cheeks flushed, he still managed a weak smile.

"Got a present for you," he rasped, offering up a wadded tissue. "Better put on a glove first."

How could he have gotten so much worse since she left him? She felt the same panic rising that she saw in Nate's face. True, Nick hadn't responded all that well to the amphotericin B—it had taken two rounds of the antifungal, but that wasn't uncommon. It could take months, she knew, to knock out a case of histoplasmosis, and then it might quickly return. But he'd been holding his own and managing all the symptoms pretty well. What was going on? She opened the tissue.

"Oh no," she whispered, looking from the rust-colored sputum in the tissue to Nick's exhausted face.

"TB," he said.

"Your X-rays didn't show TB, though," she reasoned. "We confirmed the Histo—and it was responding to the antifungal treatment. Maybe you've just irritated your throat so much with the coughing that you've got blood in your sputum. That could change the color."

"Avy," Nick countered weakly, "you're talking to a lab tech. I've seen this stuff before. Besides—" He was interrupted by another attack of coughing. He waved his hand weakly at Nate, who continued for him. "He's had dormant TB since he was a baby, when his father was stationed in Cuba."

Nate continued to hover over Nick, grasping his right hand, while she checked his temperature—103.7—and listened to his lungs with the stethoscope she kept in his home. Course crackles throughout, she determined, her clinical vocabulary kicking in, punctuated by these wrenching coughs. When she removed the stethoscope from her ears she caught the whine of the ambulance slowing to make the turn onto Crescent.

"Why don't you grab some of his things for a few days in the hospital," she directed Nate. She stood, and Nate gathered Nick up in a quick bear hug.

"Hey, not so hard," Nick protested. "It already feels like an elephant's sitting on my chest. I don't need to be squeezed to death by a grizzly!"

She witnessed the reluctance with which Nate released Nick. He gathered himself in resolve, pivoted, and disappeared into the

bathroom to collect some toiletries for his partner's care and comfort. Like a worried, loving spouse, she thought.

After Nick had shared his story, the characteristic that had
most defined him in her mind—that he was gay—no longer carried the weight it once had. She had come to see him as a cou-
rageous, funny, and sensitive person—someone she cared about
deeply. Clearly, Nate loved him, yet there was something about
the man that had nothing to do with his relationship with Nick,
something prickling at the edges of her consciousness, like a dream
or memory, that nagged at her. But she thrust it into a mental box
and shelved it, to be pulled out later for her to examine. Right now
she had to focus on Nick.

The ambulance made its familiar double chirp that told her it
had stopped in front of the house. Nate glanced out the window
to confirm and tossed her the leather bag holding his partner's toiletries and clothes. He swept Nick up in his arms and headed for
the stairs.

"Hey, the attendants can do that," she protested.

"I'm going to keep Niko as comfortable as I can, and it's
quicker this way," Nate responded. She followed him down the
stairs, ignoring Jessie's hostile glare at the bottom.

———————•◆•———————

Even after the siren's shriek had waned into the distance, she sat in
her car, still at the curb. It was all too much to take in. Nick was
someone who had sorted out all the conflicting pieces of his own
life and others' lives as well. She was at a loss on where to start with
her own.

In the light still pouring from the upstairs windows, the regal
white birch glowed beyond the fence. One of the trees Nick had

tended, maybe the cause of the histo infection. Recently a huge dead branch had fallen, scattering the white bark on the mulch below, reminding her of her long-ago dream—her mother buried in birch bark.

Returning to her father's home and doing this kind of work had been a sacrifice and a struggle, stripping away the toughened protection she had built around her core. The people she encountered had opened her heart to caring and tenderness, the softness she had hidden away in order to survive. Then information from her doctor hours ago had revealed her vulnerability.

Avy swallowed hard, shook herself, and squared her shoulders. Then she turned the key and the car purred to life. She pulled away from the curb with renewed purpose, determined to right herself and survive, to follow her mother's example.

Chapter 57

"I nearly did an Evel Knievel once over a little car like that one," he remarked, pointing at her Focus in the parking lot of the apartment complex.

She scrutinized the wiry little man, skin the color of the asphalt he ground up with the Harley parked before him. He sat on the seat of his walker at the edge of the parking lot, as if safeguarding the bike. He sported full black leathers down to his boots.

"On Aldridge Street?" she asked.

"Yeah! You mean it was you?"

"Well, someone on a Harley who looked remarkably like you nearly took off my front bumper last winter when I was trying to edge into traffic," she said.

"That's one of the many benefits of a bike. You can bypass all that annoying traffic backup."

"Well, right now I need to bypass *you* to visit a patient in the building." She stepped up the curb, onto the sidewalk beside him.

"Oh, yeah? You a nurse? You comin' to see LeRoy?" He shifted on the walker and rolled back a few inches to give her space.

She hesitated. Confidentiality was hard to maintain when everybody knew their neighbors' business, and clearly this guy had heard the news. LeRoy was home from the hospital and expecting company.

"Let me show you the way," he said, popping up from the walker seat and spinning it around to grasp the handles. He took off in front of her without waiting for a response and entered the building. She picked up her pace to keep up with him, led by the eagle wings emblazoned on the back of his jacket.

"Here's his apartment," he called out. "LeRoy, you in there?" He didn't wait for an answer and, before she could stop him, he had opened the door. He veered around a TV tray loaded with three remotes, a jigger of amber liquid, and a half-empty bag of pork rinds. As if riding the Harley, he weaved between an armchair and a newspaper-laden footstool and breezed past the sofa.

"Wait! Stop!" she called out, but he had disappeared into what was probably her patient's bedroom. Nonplussed at this invasion of privacy, she lingered in the doorway of the apartment, unsure if she should follow him in or back out and pretend she'd not been a part of this ambush.

Dazed, she became aware of her surroundings. The room was cluttered with Harley memorabilia, from the girlie poster on the wall to the motorcycle clock on the console table.

Her escort reentered the living room without the walker, chuckling. "Hi, I'm LeRoy. Who are you?"

Dumbfounded, her mouth hung open.

"I got ya, didn't I?"

"Are you serious?" Then she burst into laughter. "You got me, all right! So, my name is Avy, and yes, I'm here to see *you*, LeRoy!"

"Nice to meet you, Avy. But I don't need a nurse. See? I'm fine. I can take care of this stuff myself. Besides, it's temporary." "This stuff" meant his new colostomy, a brand-new opening in his gut that allowed the contents of his colon to pass into a plastic bag attached to his belly with an adhesive wafer.

Here was another client, she saw, who didn't think he needed a nurse—just like her father. Why were they always men? And why did *she* get them all? Yet she couldn't bring herself to feel angry. She was still trying to stifle her laughter.

"Well, apparently you agreed to have a nurse come visit you to teach you how to care for *this stuff*," she said.

"Well, they wanted to keep me another day and I got things to do. That was the only way they'd let me outta there."

This happened way too often, in her opinion. She was beginning to understand the dynamics between the hospitals, rehab centers, and home care. What was best for the patient was not necessarily how things turned out. She shuddered to consider what might have happened to patients she had erased from her thoughts once they left the hospital.

"Well, you're in my database," she said, pulling out her laptop, "and I'm in your apartment, so why don't we see where we go with this. Instead of my asking you all these questions, why don't you just show me that you can take care of your colostomy and I'll get out of your way."

"Now you're talking," he said and pulled his shirt loose from his leather pants.

"Hold it! Before you get all undone, where are your supplies? Let's at least make sure you have what you need before you pull everything apart. You don't want to be left without a new bag to attach."

LeRoy led her to the bathroom, where he pulled a hospital washbasin stacked with an assortment of boxes and bags from beside the toilet. Hospital discharge instructions, prescriptions, and a length of oxygen tubing spilled out as she unloaded the contents onto the countertop. A hospital towel hidden in the bottom would serve as the clean surface for the supplies.

"Okay. It looks like you've got everything you need here," she said. And a little more, she added silently. "Show me what you can do."

LeRoy's shirt came off, exposing curly gray hairs on his well-muscled chest. Above his silver Harley belt buckle, the flat edge of the colostomy wafer showed. The clock growled to life in the living room, gunning its engine twelve times to announce the time. Twelve noon. She realized she was hungry.

He made a show of unbuckling the belt, unzipped his pants, and folded back the edges of the waistband to expose the bag, bulging with air and brown goo. Under the plastic, the red mound of the colostomy stoma glistened. "Beautiful," Avy said. "Healthy, neat. You had a good surgeon."

She realized abruptly that LeRoy hadn't moved since folding back his pants. When her eyes lifted from examining the colostomy she saw his face had taken on an ashen tone.

"I think we'd better have you lie down," she said.

She maneuvered him through the doorway, holding onto his waistband in case he caved, and into his bedroom, where he collapsed on the HOG bedspread. The wings of the Harley Davidson logo outlined his stricken face.

"I guess maybe I do need some help after all," he whispered. "But from now on, could you come in through my slider? I don't want the neighbors to know."

Chapter 58

They rounded the northeast corner of the yard on their second lap, turning their backs on the fence that divided his house from the burned-out shell next door.

"Walking the perimeter," Bieger muttered.

"Hmm?"

"Walking the perimeter," the old man repeated. "That's how we got our exercise in Sagan—the concentration camp. We were allowed to walk the perimeter, inside the fence. But touching the guardrail could get you shot."

"You mentioned Sagan once before. You said there were stories."

"I don't really talk about it. It was a long time ago." He trudged on in silence.

She followed sheepishly. She regretted putting her foot through the crack of what was certainly a painful memory. The abrupt halt in their conversation allowed her to focus instead on the emerging autumn colors in the sugar maples across the street.

She had done all she could for Professor Bieger and was about to discharge him from home care. The trip around his yard, "walking the perimeter," was meant to verify that he could manage again without a cane. He never had agreed to the PT, arguing that his unsteadiness went back to the war. She was satisfied he would follow through on taking his pills, but she hated to admit defeat with the diet instructions. Would a few more visits win him over? She didn't think so. She gripped the gait belt around his waist to support him as they ascended the steps to the porch.

Once seated in his wingback, he admitted, reluctantly, that he did feel better. "Fewer headaches, and my legs don't ache like they did. For Elinore's sake, I should try to stick around."

"That's great. And I think you may be ready to graduate from Alliance. What do you think?"

"Do I get a diploma? I could hang it up next to my PhD from the U of M."

"No diploma, but you may have this pristine sheet of discharge instructions to frame and remember me by."

"Not the same at all. You know I won't forget you, and you won't be able to forget me either!" He pulled out his pipe as she pulled out the discharge paperwork. She set it on the coffee table, hesitated, then said, "I'm sorry that I woke those memories of the camp. It must have been a horrible experience." She looked away, and began to gather up her equipment to replace in the nursing bag.

"Well, I'm the one who brought it up, not you. Would you really like to hear about it? I haven't told the story in years."

"If you don't mind, I really would."

"How about some tea, then. With a beer chaser?" he teased.

"You *did* see me peek in that crock on your stove! But no thank you. I've had my protein for the day! And I still have to drive."

"I thought I was your last visit of the day."

"Yes, you are, but I have to get home in one piece." She smiled.

"Just what I like—a captive audience." He laughed and segued into his story. "Just like Sagan! That was a bona fide high culture venue. We had our own orchestra. Most of us in the camp were fly-boys, so we called it The Flying Syncopators. Wish I still had that clarinet that showed up from the Red Cross. Then there was the the-atre troupe—the Sagan Players. We performed one-act shows that we wrote ourselves. 'The Monkey's Paw.' 'The Invisible Duke.' First-run stuff! We were pretty good, too, but even if we weren't . . ." he gestured expectantly at her to complete the sentence and she responded on cue.

"Captive audience? You know, this sounds more like that old TV show, *Hogan's Heroes*. You can't tell me that being a prisoner was fun!"

"Well, we did what we could to break up the boredom and keep our sanity. It reminded us we were human and that there was a life beyond the perimeter. The head of the German YMCA donated sports equipment and instruments, but we cobbled together other things, too. And we ran two camp newspapers, 'The Stalag Stump' and the 'Kriegie Klarion.'"

Her chin jerked down as one eyebrow lifted. "What's Kriegie?"

"It was a nickname for 'flying personnel prisoners'—from the German Kriegsgefangenen—prisoners of war.

"Food parcels and mail were a rare treat. And we were allowed to write letters home—but they were censored, just like the ones coming in, and we tried to keep them cheerful for the family." His eyes sought the window overlooking the empty lot. "My Adele was not the same when I came back." He'd never spoken his wife's name before in her presence. "But then, neither was I." He shrugged off the memory and continued.

"We got cigarettes and soap as well in those Red Cross pack-ages. The Y would sometimes send movies. I'm still in love with Ingrid Bergman. Is she alive, I wonder?" For a moment his eyes glinted. "No, I believe I heard she had died from cancer. Even such a beautiful woman couldn't live forever."

Cancer. The word settled unbidden in her mind.

Elinore drifted in as usual, with tea, this time accompanied with Oreo cookies. They both reached for one. Today, Elinore's scrawny legs bore knee-high stockings gathered around her ankles, and long strings of pearls hung from her crepey neck.

Bieger continued, focused on twisting off one side of the cookie. "We could even take courses offered by other prisoners, or by mail from the Red Cross; I took algebra just to keep my mind sharp. I don't remember a bit of it anymore. And I collected the books from the Red Cross until I ran out of room." He returned his gaze to her, as if to emphasize his words and perhaps explain his ongoing collection upon returning stateside.

"By that time there were twelve of us in a room built for four. The wood-slat bunks were stacked three deep and covered in hay-stuffed burlap sacks. So, I moved the collection of books to the common room and started a lending library. From then on, all the books donated by the Red Cross went into it, as well as the ones the men finished reading—books that their families sent."

He leaned forward, as well as he could over his corpulent belly. "Where did I get the shelves, you ask?"

"Where did you get the shelves?" she asked, cooperatively.

"We learned to be resourceful. By the end of the war, our bunks were down to three slats apiece, and the wooden walls of the latrine—well—privacy was not as important as entertainment! We used everything that came into our hands and threw away nothing. Some of the men even made a short-wave radio out of Klim cans. That way we could hear the BBC and find out what was really going on outside the perimeter, instead of all the propaganda we heard inside."

"Klim cans?"

"'Milk' spelled backward. Powdered milk." He looked distastefully at the tobacco in his pipe, then dropped it into the soiled pocket of his white dress shirt and reached for the tea Elinore had set before them. "The cans came in handy for all kinds of things—cooking utensils, musical instruments, tools, little decorations. The boxes from the Red Cross became seats for our theater. Bucking the goons and making do with what we had kept us going."

She recalled Bernie's Marine mantra—improvise, adapt, overcome. It seemed a useful attitude in multiple situations.

The old man's words drifted to a stop. His hand lifted to his mouth for his pipe, but it was missing. Absently, he drew it back out of the pocket. He tilted his bulk to the left, leaning heavily against the arm of the sofa, and fumbled in his pant pocket for a worn leather tobacco pouch. He pinched out a twist of tobacco, tamped it down in his brier, and took a long time relighting it.

His mood changed, darkened, as he drew on the pipe. His words were no longer censored.

"No. Really, Sagan was terrible, in spite of what we did to stay sane," he growled around the brown teeth gripping the pipestem. "We had some fun, but the truth is we were treated like slaves— starved, frozen, and worked to death. Literally. The clothes we were issued for the German winter . . ."

He ticked them off on shaking fingers. "Four pairs of socks, three suits of winter underwear, two shirts, one pair of pants, a muffler, and a light jacket."

That could explain his clothing hoard upstairs, she realized.

"And we were allowed to wash our clothes in the concrete trough outdoors, once every two weeks. How are you supposed to wash any clothes when all you have to wear isn't enough to keep you warm?" He seemed to be arguing with the ghosts of the *stalag*. "We took turns. One guy would do the rest of his bunkmates' clothes while they shivered indoors. He'd have to wait two more weeks for his turn to get clean clothes." Again, he pointed at her with his pipestem.

"We survived by thumbing our noses at the Germans—the ferrets—with their 'secret' tunnels under the bunks to listen in on our conversations. And we lived for the occasional parcels from the Red Cross, the YMCA, or the Salvation Army, but it wasn't enough. We were still malnourished. The ferrets offered nothing but stale black bread, potatoes, kohlrabi, and maggots in the pea soup for protein." He pulled the pipe from his mouth. "We called it green death soup. Then there was its comrade, gray death soup, which was made from flour and water."

He fixed her with a stubborn glare.

"So you see, young lady, why I now choose to eat whatever I wish. If Sagan didn't kill me, diabetes is not going to. And if it does, it does."

It was the clearest dismissal Avy had ever heard. She discharged him without an argument or taking a sip of the cold tea.

Chapter 59

Two men sat on the mouse-ravaged cushions of the sofa on the porch of the run-down yellow crack house. She stepped out of the Focus, waved to Fred, and headed up the familiar walk. Sycamore leaves—the same dull yellow as the house—scuttled across the sidewalk in her path. The summer humidity had dissipated and a teasing fall breeze tugged at her skirt.

"Who's your friend?" she called.

"Friend? I caught him jaywalking and made a citizen's arrest!"

The other man, stretched out full length with his hands cupping the back of his neck, released one hand to deliver a punch to Fred's right shoulder with a grin.

"The guy seems to know him, although I can't imagine how," she muttered.

"Hey, bro, you've forgotten your manners!" he said.

He leveraged himself out of the sofa, towering—like Fred—over Avy. His hand stretched out and engulfed hers in a strong grip.

"I'm Jay," he said. "Fred's baby brother." He turned and kicked Fred's worn shoe. "I haven't heard that dumb 'jaywalking' line since you were a cop in Chicago."

To someone who didn't know him, Fred's eyes threatened imminent bodily harm. "You are damn lucky, kid. That might have been my bad foot."

"That would imply you've even got a good foot to put forward!" Fred attempted to rise from the sofa, but Jay shoved him back down.

"Forgive my big brother, miss. He tries to pretend he's tough."

"Why don't you make yourself useful and go get the box of supplies for Avy," Fred said. "Then we can stay out here in the fresh air while she takes care of my foot."

"Only because you're too crippled to get it yourself," Jay responded, swinging through the door as if he belonged.

"Your brother," she said. "I thought you had no family."

"Well. Turns out I do." He shrugged.

Fred sat silently, arms crossed, avoiding her eyes like a child caught in a fib. She waited for Jay to return. She could see she wouldn't get any more information from Fred.

"Thank you," she said as Jay handed her the box.

"No problem, miss."

She unloaded the supplies as usual onto the blue pad she spread on the floor of the porch, then laid out a second to kneel on. She no longer had to soak Fred's foot in Betadine solution, instead she used a wound cleanser spray. Against all predictions, new granulation tissue was replacing the former rotted mess of his toes. He had no toenails, but she figured they might grow back eventually. Anyway, she doubted Fred would miss them. Both men leaned forward over her bent form while she pulled the drainage-soaked wrappings from Fred's foot.

"So Jay, Fred's never mentioned you." Intent on her work, she let her eyes light only briefly on his face. "What brings you here?"

His eyes, no longer jovial, met hers. "That's hard to say," he began. "It was just time to move on. And I decided to see how my brother was faring since he got sprung."

"Avy knows all about that," Fred said.

"Turns out he was worse off than I was!"

Fred huffed but made no other protest. She set down the wound cleanser and patted his skin dry with gauze. She snapped off her gloves and reached for the hand sanitizer.

"Mm-hmm." She stretched fresh gloves over her clean hands and wrapped the toes with a rope of hydro-fiber batting to soak up the drainage. Fred winced but said nothing. While she wrapped Fred's foot with layers of gauze, Jay looked into the distance somewhere between the porch railing and Chicago.

"How do you like your Focus?" he asked. "That's the first model, right?"

"It's a great car for what I need and where I am right now."

"Must have been caught in the recall, though."

"I was lucky to have my Dad's Buick to use for a few days, but I'm happy with the fix. It never gave me trouble before and doesn't now, either."

"Mind if I take a look at it?"

"I guess not." She had remembered to lock it as always. It shouldn't hurt for him to admire her baby. Jay sauntered down the steps while she finished securing the dressing.

"How long you been in town?" he called from the street. She turned to answer, but he'd become invisible. Heart pounding, she recognized the panic rising. That's a strange question to ask, she thought. And where was he? She knew nothing about the guy!

"Take it easy," Fred said, noticing her alert posture—like a deer prepared to bolt. "He's under the car." At that moment Jay rose from the far side, outlined by the setting sun. He waited for her response.

On alert, she wondered what business it was of his. Yet she answered. "Since last November." The adrenaline still raced through her blood. "I was on my way to New York, but my dad needed me here, so I stayed. Why do you ask?"

"Well, I noticed the Colorado license plate. And your skid plates look like maybe they had an encounter with something that fought back. You go off-roading in the Rockies or something?" His wide grin unnerved her, even before he said, "Did you know your bumper's scraped up?"

Of course she knew! It had happened when she'd been saved by that roadside cross. It wasn't bad enough to spend the insurance deductible to fix it. This guy was beginning to spook her. Now he was walking back up the sidewalk to the house.

"Actually, your car just brought to mind a near accident I witnessed down south a ways late last year. I think it was a car just like this one, but it was dark so I can't be sure. It was kept from rolling down the embankment by a metal cross I had erected there."

He was watching her then! But she hadn't seen a soul there that night. Her skin crawled at the thought that someone, unseen by her, must have been nearby. "Bull thistle!" She'd been in more danger than she realized. She sent a silent prayer of thanks to whoever was looking out for her.

Her body shook as she turned back to Fred and dumped the rest of the supplies back in the box, willy-nilly. She stood and hoisted her bag to her shoulder.

"It was great to be outside today, Fred—I'm loving the cooler weather, but I've got to get going, now. See you tomorrow."

"What time? If I know when you're coming, I can have the stuff out here again."

"I don't know for sure," she hedged. "It'll depend on whether another of my patients gets out of the hospital."

Jay mounted the stairs behind her, blocking her path. His mouth opened as if to say something, but she cut him off.

"Nice to meet you, Jay. You and Fred stay out of trouble now."

Jay nodded and she turned and fled down the steps, back to the safe interior of the car. She clicked the lock on impulse, headed down the street, and watched the man recede in her rearview.

"That was too weird. He was actually there. So why didn't he offer to help me?" She glanced again in her rearview. He was still standing there, watching her drive away. "Because I would have freaked out with his bulk showing up like that in the dark. Besides, I didn't need any help. I managed to get myself out of the situation." She shook her head to rid it of the strange coincidences— two in one afternoon.

Chapter 60

O nce more, her father squared off across the Scrabble board from Bieger. The professor had renewed his acquaintance with his former student and colleague, now that he was no longer her patient. Their animated conversation and competition enlivened both her father's mental state and the atmosphere of the kitchen. They were oblivious to her presence in the doorway, eating her lunch on her feet. Sweet smoke with a musty undertone wafted from their pipes. She didn't even know her father smoked, but he dipped into the Black Cavendish and tamped it down in the pipe like a pro.

Avy realized she'd had a very limited knowledge of the man she'd always called her father, but he was becoming more real to her the longer she was with him. She had done the paternity character traits test and, even without knowing her mother's blood type, it showed that he "could not be ruled out" as her father. The problem was that a Honduran man could just as easily fit those limited categories too: eye color, earlobe type, blood type. It told her nothing except that Calvin Lehrer might be her father—and might not.

The realization that "not" was just as likely set her ears ringing. She knew from her mother's journal that Calvin had not wanted children early in their marriage and that she recognized how difficult it was for him to suddenly have a family. Did she mean just taking on Auralei, or did that include her as well? As hard as it was to adopt Auralei, could he have accepted the child of a man who had raped his wife? She wondered if that was why he'd always been so distant. Jared proved that Calvin could be a loving father. Had her mother told him about the rape? The pages in the journal had been torn out. Could she ask him? No, she couldn't trust anything he said now. Most of the time he didn't even treat her as his daughter. But had he *ever* treated her as his daughter? He must have known, she concluded.

Given how he'd always treated her, she decided, *not* was the most likely.

Her childhood longing to have a different father was coming true. But be careful what you wish for, she warned herself belatedly. Now all she wanted was proof that he *was* her father, but so far, she hadn't taken the next step. It would be easy to find out with DNA testing. A mouth swab from each of them. She could manage that without a battle, and Nick would be willing to run the tests for her surreptitiously, she knew, once he was well again. But Nick was not close to well. He was still in the hospital. She hadn't been able to reach him or Nate since Saturday night.

She flipped open the phone on the second ring and her heart pounded against her ribs when she learned it was the surgeon's office.

"Your pathology results are back, Ms. Lehrer, and it's good news. As I suspected, the tumor was benign."

"It's not cancer? You're sure?"

"Yes, we're sure." Avy felt the air in the room shimmer at the words she'd waited days to hear. She breathed in relief.

"However, it was a very unusual tumor, so Doctor Nanninga requested that we send it to be further analyzed at the tumor center in Cleveland." The room receded as she choked on his words. "I want to assure you again that it is *not* malignant and we were able to excise the entire growth. You should have nothing to worry about. Your doctor will call and let you know Cleveland's findings."

What did "very unusual" mean when it related to a growth that was recently inside of her? Somewhere she'd heard the prayer, "Oh God, if I have to be sick, don't let me be an interesting case," and she'd laughed! Now she *was* one of those cases!

"Thank you," she managed to say before closing the phone. She stumbled out of the house, the two men ignoring her exit, and paused on the porch to steady herself with the railing. Bieger's ancient bicycle with its off-kilter rusted basket was chained to the stair's railing. As if anyone would steal it, she thought. Bieger— now *he's* an interesting case.

She still had patients to see, so she enclosed her new worry in a lockbox of her consciousness. She reentered her car, still warm where she had parked it only a quarter hour ago, and resumed the day's game plan. She drove into the sunshine of the Arts District downtown, hoping to find Nate's office to get an update on Nick.

Chapter 61

Bernie!"

"Hi there, darlin'!" Bernie grinned from his wheelchair, palming the tire treads to keep it in motion across the uneven brick street of the historic area of the downtown. His box of bird carvings bounced precariously on his lap. The cast was gone, but she knew Bernie enjoyed the attention he got in the wheelchair and wasn't *about* to be seen with a walker or cane in public. He was miles from home, but she had an appointment to see him this afternoon.

"What on earth are you doing out here? How did you get here?"

"Just testing my wings! Guess I saved you a trip, angel! You can check me out right here."

"But I want to know how you got to *be* 'right here,'" she insisted, following in his wake. "And besides, I can't check you out here. All our supplies are at your house."

"Oh, all right. I hitched a ride with Nathan. He works at an office somewhere around here and I wheeled a ride. I was going stir-crazy up on that hill by myself."

"You never said he had an office job. I thought he just did odd jobs for Arnie."

"I don't know what all he does besides that." His brow furrowed. "He never lived with me and Rowena, so I guess I really never took the opportunity to find out what he did or who he worked for."

"So he just dropped you off in the middle of the street?"

"No, of course not!" Bernie waved off the absurd question. "On the corner there." He shot a thumb over his shoulder. "Just before you came along."

"And how are you supposed to get home?"

"He said he just had a few things to do that would keep him busy for a couple hours. He'll pick me up from the diner down the block. I finally get to ratchet-jaw with my old buddies."

"Oh, Bernie!"

"Besides, I wanted to deliver my LBJs in person to Cari, here." They stopped in front of a boutique called Flights of Fancy. "She likes me." He winked up at her. She saw a lanky brunette, dressed in flowing indigo, through the shop window.

Birdsong greeted her as she held the door open for Bernie.

"I never saw you," Avy warned him, arching an eyebrow at his grinning face, "but I'm hurt that you would choose her company over mine. I'll be at your place around 3:00 and you'd better be back in that La-Z-Boy."

She left Bernie, who wheeled through the entry, calling, "Hi darlin'!"

This gave her a little more time to track down Nate, she reasoned. She knew his architectural firm was down here somewhere. She just had to find it in the maze of diagonal streets. She recrossed the red brick road to lock her car, cut down a side street, and there it was. "Bless my navigation genes," she muttered, opening the heavy glass door.

The interior of the office space contained several sterile-looking cubicles. Beyond the etched glass of the nearest one, she recognized Nate standing at a drafting table, cell phone to his ear. His unruly hair was pulled back in a neat ponytail. Again, he was pacing. Did he ever stand still?

The phone snapped back onto his belt and he strode out of the cubicle. She stepped back and grabbed his elbows to steady him as he stumbled into her.

"Oh, I'm so sorry! I didn't see you there," he exclaimed.

"I stopped by to see how Nick is doing. I didn't know your number," she said.

Nate shook his head as if to clear his thoughts, sighed deeply, and steered her by the shoulder out the door with him. "I don't know if I'm glad to see you or not. Sorry," he said. "That came out wrong. I've got enough going on for two people." He laughed humorlessly, then stopped short and studied her puzzled face.

"You haven't figured it out, yet, have you?"

"I'm not sure I know what you mean. I know you and Nick—"

"That's not what I mean. I know you're not stupid," he said. "I'm going to have to make this fast. I'm sorry. And I could use your help, too, if you're willing."

"Yeah, if I can. I'm working, though. I just stopped by hoping to catch you here and find out about Nick."

"Okay. Here's the condensed version. Nick is in isolation, not doing well. And Mrs. Berndt's daughter just called me. We have until Friday to find new quarters. She was 'appalled'—punctuated with cringing and hand-waving—to find that her mother had let a couple of queers rent *her* old space upstairs. Meanwhile I'm camping out at my dad's house, but"—he filled his lungs and rushed on—"he doesn't know I'm gay."

She swallowed all other questions except "How do you think I can help?"

"I brought him into town with me, but Dad needs a ride back home, because I have to head to the hospital now. Can you take him? I think you were planning to come out to the house anyway today."

Her head was spinning. Her thumb and third finger pressed her temples and she squinted up at Nate's face. "That's it," she said. "That's what puzzled me the other night. You're Bernie's stepson, Nathan."

"Bingo," he said. "Only Niko—Nick to you—calls me Nate." Avy nodded dumbly. "Can you take Bernie home without looking like a concrete block has just fallen on your head? I know I have to tell him, but now is just not the time. And it needs to come from me."

"Yeah," she said, still trying to fit all the puzzle pieces in place. "Yeah, I'll take him home. I just ran into him crossing the road. Um, I need to see another patient first, and then I can meet him at the diner where he'll be kibitzing with his buddies." She fished in her purse for a pen. "Here's my cell number," she said, writing on the back of a business card. Will you call me when you get a chance and let me know what's happening with Nick?"

Nate pulled her into a spontaneous hug. "You bet. Thanks. You're a godsend."

On her way home from Bernie's, Avy programmed the GPS for the nearest drugstore. She had returned home from work twice to the odor of feces and a boggy spot on the sofa that her father had tried to clean up. The first time she believed his explanation that it was Alex who had made the mess. Maybe her father believed that, himself. Alex had outlived the average lifespan for a fox terrier by

several years. He was going deaf and nearly blind; it was natural he
would begin to lose control of his bowels too. But the second time
it happened, she found her father's soiled pants in the recycle bin.

Avy had never bought Depends and didn't know how she
could get her father to accept them, but it had to happen. Standing
there, she was more embarrassed than when she had started buying her own menstrual supplies. She moved to the end of the aisle
to think. In front of her was a display of a variety of home tests
for everything from pregnancy to steroids. And paternity. A home
DNA test for paternity? It made buying the Depends much less
embarrassing.

Chapter 62

Avy had left the kitchen table to answer her phone. Her father pushed the Mongolian beef around on his plate, scowling. Dr. Nanninga had discouraged the Hunan chicken as contributing to his "dyspepsia." Avy was trying to introduce a milder item from the Chinese takeout menu. Her father was getting as picky as a two-year-old about his food. Distracted by her father's displeasure, she missed what the voice on the phone was saying.

"I'm sorry?" she asked.

"Niko," said the strained voice she now recognized as Nathan's. "He died a few hours ago."

"No! Oh, Nathan. I'm so sorry." Behind her, a fork clattered on the tile. The scrape of a chair sliding across the floor caused her to glance over her shoulder. Her father held his plate inches off the floor, where Alex greedily devoured the treat.

"The official cause of death will be TB so I can blame it on his father and his military career." A bitter edge cut through the last word. "The family has been informed by the hospital. They were apparently relieved that Niko had a living will naming me as DPOA. They won't have to be involved."

Her father cracked open a fortune cookie. "Grief is the price we pay for love," he read slowly, then announced, "Your lucky numbers are 6, 14, 39, 56 and 72."

"Where are you, Nathan? What can I do?" she asked.

"I'm just leaving the hospital now. I have to go over to the funeral home in the morning to make arrangements." He hesitated. "This is such an imposition. You hardly know me, but would you be willing to meet me there? I don't think I can do this alone."

"Yes, of course," Avy said, mentally rearranging her schedule. "What about tonight? Are you going back to Bernie's?"

"Avy, I haven't told him anything. He doesn't know about Niko. How can I just walk back in the house after this and act normal?"

"Hey, we've got an extra room here in my dad's house. You can stay with us." Part of her brain was objecting even as she blurted out the invitation. What was happening to her? She had just breached her own boundary fence, not to mention the complete lack of professionalism it revealed.

"No. That's a generous offer, but I'm not going to be any good around people for a while. I need to be alone for now. I'll get a hotel."

"I understand, but call me if you need anything before we meet tomorrow morning. I'm here."

———— ◆ ————

At 10:00 a.m. Nathan, looking as if he hadn't slept at all, held the door open for her and they entered the dimly lit interior of the funeral home. He took her hand for support and she gave it a brief squeeze. She sat breathing quietly beside him as the funeral director verified Nathan's authority to make the arrangements for cremation and to take possession of the cremains. Then he slid several thick binders in front of them to choose an urn. After flipping through them all, Nathan chose a walnut box inlaid with a teak carving of a weeping willow shading a tranquil stream. "Niko loved nature," he said.

They exited into the daylight. As they reached her car, she ignored her internal censor.

"Nathan, are you sure you're okay staying at a hotel? Did you sleep at all last night? It would really be fine for you to stay with us. Think about it. Maybe stop by for dinner tonight at least."

"You know, I think I might take you up on dinner. I thought I wanted to be alone, but it just opens up this huge emptiness where Niko used to be." He ran fingers through his loose blond curls and shook his head. "And, no, I didn't get much sleep last night. But your kindness and support has been so helpful. What time is dinner?"

"Can you be there by 5:30? Dad needs to eat early. And I make a mean spaghetti."

"I'll be there."

She climbed into the Focus, his hand under her elbow for support. He leaned in and touched his forehead to hers with a sigh.

"Thank you," he managed. Instinctively, she kissed his cheek before he could step away.

"Avy, you're an angel. I don't know how to thank you for everything you've done to help me already."

"It's my pleasure. See you tonight."

―――――――――⋯ ◆ ⋯―――――――――

Her father had taken to Nathan at dinner that night, although she couldn't guess what he might understand about why he was there. Nathan seemed to have a natural ability to engage her father in a way that was respectful and affirming, despite the raw grief that filled him, and her father had responded. Then after dinner, when he had absented himself to his office, they made plans.

"I'll be seeing Bernie again tomorrow afternoon around 3:00," she said. "I can stay if you want support to talk to him then," she offered.

"I need to get this over with sometime," he said. She waited for his decision, and he pressed his lips together before responding. "If I come when you're still there, it means I'm ready. But if I don't come it means I couldn't face him yet. Okay?"

"Either way. I've got your back. I'm just glad you've agreed to stay here with us for a bit." He stifled a yawn. "C'mon, let's get you settled."

Chapter 63

A vy pulled into Bernie's driveway at 3:00 on Monday. She wondered if Nathan would have the courage to follow through with the tentative plan they had made, if he was ready to tell Bernie that he was gay.

"Nathan was sleeping here lately," Bernie said, as if reading her mind. "He said it gave him more time to work on the bathroom in the evenings, but I think something else is going on. Now he hasn't been around for a couple of days, and he never let me know he wasn't coming back," he said as Avy redressed the pressure ulcer that had developed under the cast. By the time the cast had been removed it was a stage 3 and should take at least a month to heal completely. Bernie was expected to do the daily care himself, but Avy was convinced from the look of it on her weekly visits that he skipped more than a day or two. Not that he'd ever admit it.

"It seems like it would make sense that he stays here while he's working on the bathroom," she agreed, applying the Silvadene cream to the wound with sterile gauze. The pressure sore was healing more slowly than she had expected. She considered increasing the frequency of her visits to ensure it was being attended to as it should be.

Bernie said nothing while she fluffed more gauze into his wound, wrapped it snugly with stretch gauze, and sealed the end with tape. As she pulled a clean tube sock over the dressing, Bernie continued.

"Nathan was already out of the house when Rowena married me, but I do love the boy and I really would like to have a closer relationship with him. He's been very good to me, and I like having him around, but he always seems to hold something back. Until a few days ago, he had never stayed here overnight. Then, without a word, he just disappeared again." He scrunched up his face in a puzzled frown. "I don't know if I did something to set him off or what."

"Family relationships can be complicated, I know, Bernie," she said, settling into a chair at his side.

"No lie." He shrugged and turned to her. "I wish he had enough faith in me to just come out and say whatever's eating him." She leaned toward him, her hands open in her lap. He hesitated, but decided he could trust her. "He'd have every reason to think I'd be disgusted. I've shot off my big mouth often enough, but I'm pretty sure he's—"

"Gay, Bernie," Nathan said, leaning on the doorjamb. "A faggot, a queer, a fairy. How many more pejoratives have I heard come out of your mouth for men like me?" He dragged another dining room chair into the room and dropped into it, a few inches from where Avy sat, a buffer between the two men. "How could I come out to you?"

Bernie was silent for a good ten seconds. Then he said, "I guess I made it pretty hard, didn't I?"

Nathan sat forward, lips parted as if to speak, but instead his face twisted and he reached for Avy's hand. His hand in hers was cold and moist. "Would you tell him the rest?" he asked.

She squeezed his hand in affirmation, then turned her eyes from him and studied Bernie's. His face registered the weary resignation of having his suspicions confirmed, and confusion that she seemed to know all about it. His face twitched as he sat with the information.

He gathered himself together and forced his elevated leg to the floor, away from Nathan's outstretched hand resting in hers—the hand that had just gently cleaned and dressed his ulcer and that was apparently comfortable holding the hand of a stepson who might be contaminated with a horrible virus.

"You've got AIDS," Bernie said.

She dropped Nathan's hand and reached for Bernie's, but he folded his arms across his chest, closing himself off. She sensed his hurt but not that she was part of the cause. Still, she was determined to fulfill Nathan's request.

"No, Bernie, not AIDS." She held her gaze kindly on Bernie's shrouded eyes, which looked right past her, out the window, toward the plaster saint down the hill. And the rest of her words drifted to the floor between them like the russet leaves coasting down outside the window.

Bernie let the two of them leave without a word in response.

Chapter 64

Avy's throbbing head rested on the back of the driver's seat. The headrest grazed her damp crown. The headaches had been coming more often lately, ever since her concussion, but she hadn't had a migraine like this for months. Lights flashed like fireworks bursting on the background of her closed lids.

She hoped she could just get into the house and into bed before her stomach got into the act.

She groped for the door handle, but before she was able to lift her head from the headrest, the door swung outward. Her eardrums reverberated with the squeal of the hinges. She dragged one eye half-open. Nathan peered in at her, the sun behind his head threatening to lance through her brain if he moved an inch.

"I hoped he was with you."

"Who—Bernie?" she whispered.

"No, your dad. He and Alex were both gone when I got here a few minutes ago."

Her eyes flew open and quickly shut again, her brain now torn in two like a walnut split down its sulcus. "Spurge!" she whimpered.

Head held in her cupped hands, she asked, "Nathan, can you help me get inside? I'm afraid I'm going to barf."

She felt herself lifted gently from the driver's seat. Behind her the door closed with the sound of a steel drum. Cradled in Nathan's arms, she floated over the grass and up the two steps. She rocked gently as he carried her upstairs to her room.

She heard the swish of the window blinds lowering. "I've put your wastebasket on the floor here by your head in case you need to throw up. I'm going to get a cold cloth. I'll be right back."

"Mmhm."

She was vaguely grateful that for once Alex wasn't barking. She couldn't remember what Nathan had said about the dog. Whatever it was, it could wait.

Nathan returned with the cloth for her forehead. "I'll leave your door open a crack. I'll hear if you need me. I'm right down the hall. Just rest." His gentle voice comforted her just as her mother's voice used to—or was it her father's voice? Tears leaked from under Avy's fragile lids. She slept.

———◆———

"Trust the wings."

Her mother's voice. Avy observed with curiosity the naked woman on the floor and wondered if she was dead. No, an eye had opened, but she looked as if she might not live long. Avy would watch and wait. There was nothing else to do.

She felt a wave of nausea as the woman rolled her head stiffly on the tile floor and opened the other eye. She watched the lashes pull away from the skin of the woman's hopeless face. Her mother's face.

"Trust the wings."

Avy felt impossibly heavy, her limbs incredibly weak. Her body sank back into the cold darkness of sleep.

——•——

Insistent barking pierced the blue-black ink of her consciousness and she woke once more. Alex flung himself onto her bed, lapping at her sweaty face. She rolled to her side and vomited into the wastebasket. Footsteps thundered up the stairs. A frantic scolding urged, "Alex, get out of there! Come!" She rolled sluggishly back onto the damp sheets and tentatively cracked open one eye. Nathan had collared Alex and handed him off to her father standing in the doorway. Another form hovered behind him.

"Smells a bit like green death soup in there," a familiar gruff voice said. "Nurse, heal thyself!"

"Let me get rid of this and I'll be back." Nathan laid the cloth that had covered Avy's forehead over the top of the wastebasket and shut the door behind him. She heard her father drop Alex on the hardwood floor of the hallway and shuffle off, grumbling to Professor Bieger.

She wondered if she could still be dreaming, and thought she heard her mother's voice again, far away.

"Trust the wings."

Avy hooked one bare foot over the edge of the bed until, by propping herself on her left elbow, she could touch the rug with her toes. The thunder in her head had softened like a storm wearing itself out after it blew by. Nathan returned just as she rose, swaying, and he held out a warning hand.

"You've been out for about three hours. Are you feeling well enough to be up?"

"Not sure," she said, sinking back onto the bed, remembering the dream. "Am I hallucinating or did I hear Dr. Bieger in the hall?"

"Apparently, he decided to pay a visit to your father this afternoon. He brought his own Scrabble set this time as he realized your dad's set was missing some letters. They've been locked in battle ever since they got back from walking the dog."

"Walking the dog? Dad never takes Alex out of the yard."

"Well, I guess he didn't remember that. Alex took them on quite a trek by all accounts! Once past the fence, he took off. Luckily, he's attracted to Saltines. Old Bieger had a pocketful, and Alex followed the trail of crumbs like Hansel till they got him home. That was just a few minutes after you conked out."

"What would I have done if you hadn't been here?"

"Probably passed out on the front lawn and been licked to death by your crazy dog." She tried to smile.

Nathan rolled her desk chair over to the bed. "Now is not the time to worry about it, but you and I both know that your father's going to need more care than you can give."

Her father often wandered around the house late at night now. She was grateful Nathan slept lightly and got up to hold midnight conversations with him, during which they drank schnapps and ate Pecan Sandies.

"I know!" she whimpered. "I just don't know what to do!" She always knew exactly what to do, she thought, but now . . .

"Hey, you need to rest and get your head back on straight. Meanwhile, trust me, I'll be here."

"Trust me," she thought. "Trust the wings." Trust had never come that easy. But what choice did she have? Trusting, she rolled back onto her side and slept.

Chapter 65

She checked the website for the fourth time. And this time her case number appeared in the list. The DNA results were in. She logged off quickly, heart pounding, without entering her private ID number for the answers.

As she drove downtown, her troubled eyes took in the few brown and yellow leaves left on the oaks and birches. Lawns were already awash in the vibrant reds, oranges and golds of the maples. Unconsciously, she smiled at the palette she had missed in Denver. The aspens there just went to yellow in autumn. Yellow wasn't her color. She detoured to Robinson Road. Yes! Here the deep cranberry-wine leaves of the sumacs still held their color, fed by the swampy verge of an unnamed feeder creek that trickled into the lake. Bare oak trunks leaned haphazardly above the sumacs, proof they didn't belong where the sumacs thrived.

"Where do I belong? Am I like sumac or oak? Maple or birch?"

Her closest friend was a gay man who had moved seamlessly into her father's home and life in a matter of days. Nathan was the perfect companion to her father in their odd household. Their mutual interests in history and architecture supplied a foundation of conversation and gateways of respect between her friend and her father. He had not had such a knowledgeable companion since his retirement, and now he had two. Bieger was a regular visitor, bringing stale Saltines and Scrabble.

She found a parking spot a few blocks from the farmers' market. The spring greens had long ago been replaced with the last of the summer tomatoes and the fall squash, apples and sunflowers. She recognized the dried wildflowers that had bloomed with all the shades of spring. She chose a bunch of hyssop—still muted purple—and a cheesecloth bag of lavender buds tied with twine. She held the bag to her nostrils and breathed in the calming fragrance. When she opened her eyes, she noticed a small crowd pressed around an orchard booth touting a new apple variety, grown and available locally only from this one orchard—*Kryst!* The farm where she had purchased the "aspergrass" last spring. She craned her neck over the crowd, but the booth was managed by a middle-aged woman, not the youth she had met on her first trip to Bernie's place. Avy hadn't seen Bernie now for almost a week. She wondered how he was doing. She got in line for a sample of the new Gold Rush apple and found it sweet and spicy with a hint of citrus—perfect for fall. She bought a half peck.

"Avy?" She whirled with her bag of apples to look for the source of the greeting.

"Claire!" She hadn't seen Claire since she'd rescued Joyce and her boys from the old farmhouse. As they broke apart from a warm hug, Avy admired the flowing fall colors of Claire's tunic. "You are clearly a fall person," she said.

"I won't deny it. I love this time of year."

"I was just ready to head back to the car, but I wonder if you have a few minutes to talk."

"I was going back to my office, but I'd rather enjoy the outdoors a while with you. We could sit in the churchyard if you like."
They ambled companionably up the block to the church where
they'd first met. "Why don't you pick a spot. I need to get these
flowers in water before they wilt. I'll be right back."

She found a concrete bench in a copse of trees. Sitting, she let her
mind wander. It returned to the website that held the results of the
paternity test. She had shut it down without learning the truth. Just
then, her cell phone rang, insistently repeating until she answered.

"Miss Lehrer?" She recognized the voice of her doctor's receptionist. "Dr. Nanninga would like to have you come in Monday
to discuss the tumor findings with him. Can you come at noon?"

"It's cancer after all, isn't it?"

"You'll need to discuss it with him, I'm afraid. But he did ask me
to reassure you that it was *not* a malignancy." Avy blew out a breath.

"I can make it," she said, and ended the call. So, she wondered,
what awful thing could have invaded her body, then? If the growth
was not a malignancy, then what? Some kind of parasitic worm?

"I brought us some iced tea." Claire's voice carried across the
courtyard to where Avy sat numbly on the bench. She looked up as
the woman drew near.

"Something has changed," Claire said. "I heard your phone
ringing. Did you receive some bad news?"

"Yes and no. I don't know what to think."

"Would you like to talk about it?"

"I don't know where to start. I used to know who I was. Now
everything about me is a muddle."

"I'm in no hurry. Let's unmuddle you a bit if we can."

Chapter 66

She had never felt so reluctant to face a patient she enjoyed. Especially Bernie. She stopped her car beside the mailbox. Maybe another stroll in Rowena's garden will clear my head, she thought. She glanced up the hill through the dusty haze. Was he watching her? Should she say anything at all or just go on as if nothing has changed? She moved toward the dried edge of the flower thicket, kicking up more dust with her new suede boots. The entrance to the labyrinth eluded her. The touch-me-nots had given way to a bright flurry of black-eyed Susans, white asters, and late-season sunflowers. Too cheery for her mood. She looked down at her new boots, covered in dust, and turned back toward her car.

"Looking for me?" Bernie's head cropped up among the nodding yellow blooms.

"Everlasting pea!" she squealed. "Why did you do that?"

Bernie gulped air, laughing until hiccups took over. "I didn't mean to scare you," he said. "Wasn't even thinking about how you'd take to such a hulk rising out of the sunflower patch."

Avy couldn't help it. She leaned against her car, her hands pressing on her galloping heart, and laughed her relief. Bernie climbed onto the driveway and dropped his three-fingered paw on her shoulder.

"Hold me up while I bend over to stop these confounded hiccups."

She grabbed him by a belt loop. "I should let you fall on your bald head and knock some sense into you." A minute later, he blew out a heaving breath, swung upright, and grinned at her.

How could she not want to see Bernie?

"Well, if you can squeeze yourself into the passenger seat, I'll give you a ride to the top."

In fifteen minutes she had finished redressing his leg ulcer. It was coming along in spite of his admitted neglect of the daily dressing changes. She bagged up the old wrappings to throw into his trash.

"So, how's Nathan?" he asked then. "Have you seen him lately?"

"Actually, he's been staying with me and my father. I know he'd like to move on and get his own place, though."

"Do you think he'd be willing to see me? I'd like to talk with him. I've had a long time to try to sort out my feelings, but I'm not getting very far. I think I need to go to the source. I need to listen to him like you have."

"That's always a good idea," she agreed. "I'll give you my home number. If he's not at work, that's where he'll likely be. Call him."

"Thanks, honey. You've been—well, I don't know how to tell you what you've been to me and to my son. An angel, I'd say! I was upset last week, but the problem was with me, not you. Besides, I couldn't be angry with you for long."

Very unprofessionally, she kissed the top of his bald head. As she had kissed the top of her father's head upon leaving that morning. Her *true* father, Calvin Lehrer.

Chapter 67

"Avy, thank you for meeting with me today." Dr. Nanninga shook her hand. His face wore a bemused look. With his brows scrunched together, his smile was thin, hiding his teeth. "Please have a seat." She obeyed.

"As I told you before, the tumor we removed was *not* a malignant cancer. Yet neither the surgeon nor I had ever seen anything like it. I didn't want to frighten you any more than you already were, so I had it analyzed, and the Cleveland staff was excited when they realized what it was."

Avy nodded tersely. She felt somehow violated by the number of people examining a private part of her body that *she* hadn't even seen and didn't understand.

The doctor continued. "What we removed was a teratoma. These are quite rare, hence the excitement in Cleveland." He waited, as if he expected her to ask a question, but Avy could only think of a similar word, tarantella—a wild folk dance—and envisioned whatever this thing was quickstepping pain up and down her spine.

He went on. "A teratoma goes by several other names: dermoid cyst, fetus in fetu, or parasitic twin." She tried to concentrate, but now she saw twin *fetuses* whirling around.

"Fetus? I had a fetus in my back? That's impossible! It makes no sense at all."

"That's part of the problem. We don't fully understand how these tumors develop. There are several theories. Do you know if twins run on your mother's side in your family?"

"Not as far as I know. My mother had a younger sister, not a twin."

"One theory is that at the time of conception, two eggs are fertilized, either by one sperm or two. They both begin to grow side by side into fetuses. If one of these twin fetuses is stronger—most likely the older one—it's surmised that the underformed twin becomes absorbed into the stronger, and only one will grow to full maturity. The other can't survive, except as a parasitic cyst. This is what we found in you."

"You're saying *I* had a twin?"

"Not a *viable* twin, but yes, your twin was absorbed into you. We might have found it anywhere, or never known it was there, but because it pressed against your spine, causing pain, we looked there."

A parasitic twin, like an invasive species, that she'd been carrying around all this time. Her mind reeled in its own wild dance.

"There was another finding that makes your case unique," he said. "Your blood type and DNA are different from that of the tumor. This would indicate you had two different biological fathers—or sperm donors might be a more accurate way to say it."

She began to giggle.

Dr. Nanninga's face crumpled in surprise. "Avy! Are you all right? Do you understand what I'm telling you?"

"Two days ago I didn't know which of two men was my father. Yesterday I got the results from a paternity test and found out I wasn't a bastard after all. The man I always knew as my father was in fact that. Today you tell me I've been carrying a bastard fetus around with me wherever I go. Part of me." She shook her head. "It will take a little while for me to grasp this fully, but I do understand what you've said. Yes." She wiped her eyes with a tissue. Then, "You're sure they got it all, right?"

"Yes, Avy. They got it all."

Chapter 68

Ms. Lehrer?"

"This is Aviana Lehrer. How can I help you?"

"This is Kathleen Post from the Lenten House. Joyce Quinlan gave me your number and asked that I call you. I wonder if you'd be willing to meet with me and Joyce this week. Her time here is running out and she's been unable to locate a safe place for herself and her children. We'd like your input on some options we've talked about."

"I don't know how I can help you. I was involved with Joyce only because I was the home care nurse for someone in her family." She hadn't given much thought to the young woman after she'd gotten her and her sons into the Lenten House several months ago. The few times the Quinlan family had crossed her mind, the phrase "white trash" appeared like a headline in her thoughts. She'd gone out of her way, and maybe even put herself in danger, to get them to safety. It was not her way to become involved with people like this.

"I'm working full-time and my father requires a lot of care in the evening, so I don't know when I could meet with you."

"Yes, I know. Joyce has told me all about how you saved her grandmother's life."

"Well, that may be a bit of an exaggeration. I was just doing my job. If I'd been more observant, I might have gotten her grandmother out of there sooner and never seen Joyce again. I wouldn't have gotten involved, except maybe I needed closure. I don't know what more I can do."

She heard only empty silence at the other end of the line. She recalled Joyce's spunk, and her desperation to get away from the consequences of what she had seen and done. Despite herself, she smiled at the memory. Joyce had gained some self-esteem while caring for her grandmother. She recognized the feeling.

"Wait—Kathleen, is it?" She expected that Nathan would be at the house tonight. She would call him to be sure. "I don't really know what I could contribute, but I could probably stop by right after work—around 4:30?"

"That would be great," Kathleen said. "We're just brainstorming and not coming up with a good solution, so anything you could add would help. We'll see you this afternoon."

She ended the call and resumed documenting the previous visit she had made. She found herself becoming increasingly involved in other people's lives—other people's problems. She had enough of her own. Which brought her father to mind. She dialed Nathan's cell.

"Nathan Thorne."

"Hi, Nathan. It's Avy."

"Hey, Avy! I was just thinking of you. I've got an idea to run by you, but I thought I'd wait till you got home. I'm planning to make goulash if that sounds good."

"It's great if you can hold it till about 6:00. I just made a commitment that will take me some time this afternoon and I wanted to check if you'd be able to keep an eye on my father till I got home."

"Not a problem. He can help me cook."

"Great! So do I get a hint of this idea of yours?"

"Nope. Focus on what you have to do and we'll talk over goulash. Six it is."

Chapter 69

Avy had succeeded so far in blocking out a thought that had tried to invade her mind during the meeting. It was just not feasible. Her boundaries had already been breached repeatedly in the past year since she had left Denver. Her mind guarded this section of its fence like a border patrol, determined to prevent any more illegal crossings.

At least she could relax for a few days. It was Monica's turn to work the weekend and she would see Fred. He'd taken a liking to Monica when she had seen him during Avy's surgery.

She could smell the goulash before she opened the door. Her internal border patrol stood at ease.

"Perfect timing," Nathan said as she entered the kitchen. Her father was already at the table, pouting with impatience. Alex was stationed beside his chair, ready to pounce on any stray tidbits. She shucked her lab coat in the laundry room and washed her hands in a sink full of cooking pots.

"I could get used to coming home to your cooking," she said with a sigh.

"Wait till you've tasted it. You might change your mind."

"The smell tells me I won't. Is this how you plan to soften me up for your big idea?"

"That would be much too devious for my simple mind." He winked. "But if it works . . ." One by one, Nathan placed steaming bowls of goulash on the table. A basket of fresh bakery bread graced the center. Her father picked up his spoon.

"Hold on, Cal. It's too hot yet. You'll burn your tongue," Nathan warned. "You could start with a piece of bread if you want." Her father obediently laid his spoon down at Nathan's suggestion and snatched a piece of bread instead. She slid into her usual spot by the window and reached for a chunk as well. She wondered how this had become normal.

"Okay, so what's this idea of yours?"

Nathan chewed on his piece of bread. His eyes shifted toward her father and back to her. He obviously didn't want to talk about it in front of him.

"Tell me about your day first," he countered.

"The students are getting stupider every year," her father said. "Today, I graded the papers on Homer and not a single one made any sense. I'm going to have to fail the lot of them." He plunged his bread into the goulash with a vengeance, sloshing globs onto the Formica tabletop. Alex whined with impatience.

"That's a shame," Nathan said. "You work so hard on your lectures. It must be terribly frustrating to have such thickheaded students."

"At least someone understands what I have to put up with," Calvin said. "I spoke with the dean and he's just as clueless as the students. I don't know if I can hold out until retirement. My colleagues tell me it's just as bad for them. Old Bieger says he retired just in time."

Avy joined in. "How's Professor Bieger doing?"

Her father grinned. "I can still beat him in Scrabble. His mind isn't as sharp as it used to be. He misses the most obvious words."

"Well, maybe you should take it easy on him." She recalled the fierce Scrabble competitions she had endured with her father.

"Easy? What would be the point in that? If you can't play an honest game, you shouldn't play. If I ease up, he'll never learn to play well."

She had learned to play so well against her father that her opponents over the years had dropped out of her life. "Anything worth doing is worth doing right" was the mantra drilled into her in her youth. It had driven her all of her life. If you can't be the best, you're not trying hard enough. If you can't win, don't play. And if someone gets the job you thought was yours, leave. And end up here, back where you started, she realized.

The table cleared, Nathan poured two glasses of Riesling—Old Mission, her favorite. He tipped his head toward the living room. She checked that her father had slipped away to his study, ostensibly to grade more papers.

"You *are* trying to soften me up," she said, sprawling into the ugly, but comfortable, pumpkin-orange chair in the living room. "And after the day I've had. My brain's on empty and I'm fresh out of ideas for myself, so I'm ready to hear yours." She took a large gulp of the wine.

"Don't drink too much of that at once! I don't want to have to carry you upstairs again."

"Just tell me you've solved the mystery of my life and I'll go along with anything."

"Solving the mystery of your life is up to you, but this crazy idea may help along the way somehow—maybe." He stopped and set down his wine glass, untouched. "Nah. Who am I kidding?

Maybe I'm just being selfish. I've got nothing to lose, though, so here goes."

She set her glass on the floor and sat up straighter.

"I've practiced saying this until I could make it come out right. But now it sounds pretty lame."

Her gut clenched. He looked so insecure, but hopeful. She was afraid to hear what he was thinking.

"You know that house that Niko and I lived in? It's up for sale. Mrs. Berndt's daughter has moved her into an assisted living facility. It was already settled when she arrived that awful day. She had contacted a realtor, and made the arrangements without even consulting Tilda. That was another reason she kicked us out so abruptly. She planned to get it cleaned out and listed while she was there, and I'm sure she had the entire upstairs where we lived fumigated. What a horrible woman, so different from Tilda."

She couldn't disagree. How sad for Mrs. Berndt, she thought.

"So. My crazy thought is that I want to live there again, where Niko and I were happy together."

"What?" This was not what she had just begun to fear. "And how does this involve me?"

"Unfortunately, I don't have enough cash for a down payment and I wouldn't want to take on a loan right now with interest rates so high. Besides, Jessie would never sell it to me anyway. As soon as she saw my name on the offer, that would be the end of it." He rushed on. "But, I thought maybe, if I was willing to make a long-term commitment, you might think about buying it and I could rent from you. You and your dad could live there on the main level and I could still help you with him in the evening. It's in walking distance from Dr. Bieger's house and he could continue to visit." Nathan stopped, his face reflecting both hope and anxiety.

She sat stunned, a throbbing pulse building behind her eyes. "Whew."

"Oh, Avy, I'm sorry I even brought it up. I *am* being selfish. Forgive me. Drink your wine."

She reached absently for the glass on the floor.

"What would make you think *I* had that kind of money?" Her right index finger circled the rim, eliciting a faint wail that she seemed not to notice. "Besides, I never planned to stay long in Berndtbridge."

Silence fell between them. From her father's study a continuous mixture of disgruntled mumbling, punctuated by chair legs scraping wood, provided a background.

She never planned to stay in Berndtbridge, yet here she was a year later. The rules of the game had changed when she wasn't paying attention.

She sat slumped, eyes cast down to the floor. Original hardwood, she thought to herself. Lifting her head, she also noted the ample light entering the picture window at sunset. And the attractive wooden trim and stair railing.

"Give me the realtor's info," Avy said. "I've got an idea of my own."

Chapter 70

"No running on the stairs!" Joyce called out. Four-year-old Reid, scuttling down from the upstairs apartment, ignored her. Avy braced herself for the expected verbal explosion, but heard only, "Did your kids ignore you like that when they were growing up?" In the bathroom adjoining the kitchen, Joyce held a toothbrush out to Avy's father. Avy could imagine his eyes shining on Joyce and she smiled wistfully at her own reflection in the new stainless-steel refrigerator door. No, she thought, we didn't *dare* ignore him back then.

The advancing dementia had somehow gentled her father. The family he had been unable to embrace no longer existed for him. Joyce and her boys were his family now, and Avy was only a benign presence, like a hired housekeeper, there to serve his new household. That he had been proven to be her father no longer really mattered to Avy. When little Reid said, "You have a funny thumb toe, just like Grandpa Cal's," she suddenly saw what she might have noticed years ago, if she had paid attention. Too late, she had discovered the truth of her parentage, what her parents had suffered through, the crucible that had formed them. It would still take time to completely let go of her hurt and resentment, but she was opening her heart little by little.

Following Reid, Nathan's footfalls clattered down the stairs. He whistled a tuneless snatch she vaguely recognized as he ducked through the archway on the main level and tossed a giggling Will from his shoulders into the air. He caught the boy in midair and plunked him onto the beanbag with his brother, in front of the TV where Mr. Rogers invited them into *his* living room.

Nathan would drop Reid off at preschool shortly, then meet Bernie for breakfast before checking in on his new building site on the eastern border of Berndtbridge. The two men met weekly at Jack's Joint, talking about everything, except the issue that divided them. They both liked it that way.

Bieger would arrive soon on his rattletrap bike with the Scrabble board and the day's newspaper, in time for Joyce's freshly brewed coffee and the banana bread that Avy had slid into the oven as she prepared to head out for work. Tonight she would meet Andrew for dinner at the Rock River Bar and Grill.

Avy's smile reached all the way to her eyes as she considered how her life had changed in the past year. She realized that learning her family's story had provided her a way to understand her own story, to write a new chapter that began with forgiveness, and to discover that she *did* belong—right where she was, from one day to the next. Not in striving for prestige and respect in the corporate world, like some proud, fierce, eagle, but in opening her wings to love and support her growing flock—and to receive their love in return.

The old Victorian house had opened its door to welcome all these disparate lives. As in an ordered garden giving way to wild nature, so new members had arrived in Avy's life—individuals joining in symbiosis, not as parasites or invasive species, but as a new and synergistic microcosm in which they all flourished and belonged.

"I wonder if you are the miracle you're looking for," Claire had said months back in the numinous light of the stained-glass window. Avy could begin to believe that God, *if* he existed, did work in mysterious ways. After all, if he could miraculously put words in the mouth of a stubborn donkey, maybe he could turn her into a miracle, too.

"Trust the wings," her mother had whispered from the pages of her journal and echoed in Avy's dreams. Okay, Mom, she agreed.

As she opened the door to take on another day, the crystal doorknob caught the sun's light and sprinkled an iridescent palette of colors across the heart of her white lab coat. She pulled the door shut, humming Mr. Rogers' theme song, "It's a Beautiful Day in the Neighborhood." It was. She paused on the stoop. The crisp November breeze tugged the last of the birch leaves from the ancient tree in the yard. A pair of cedar waxwings picked over the red fruit glistening on the winterberry hedge. Chipmunks scurried for those that fell to the ground. From the bare trees on the horizon, hundreds of starlings burst into a raucous chorus and ascended as one, winging across the azure sky in a murmuration dance. Her heart lifted with them as the first November snowflakes kissed her cheek.

About the Author

From crack houses to elegant mansions, dilapidated farmhouses, senior living complexes, and oncology units, Barbara Schultze followed her clients' personal stories of estrangement and reconciliation, sickness and health, and ultimately life and death. She began her nursing career as a hospital staff nurse, joined home care as a nurse case manager, rose to become a home health clinical director, and eventually became a certified hospice chaplain, listening to engrossing stories of proud military service, lost-and-found spirituality, family distress, and end-of-life joys as well as regrets.

Meanwhile, Barbara started a parish nursing program and ventured into dementia support and therapeutic riding (hippotherapy). Her chaplaincy certification included published research on using clients' tattoos to initiate meaningful conversations. She has spoken on spiritual care in end-of-life situations, and was featured on the cover of *HomeCare Expert Coding* magazine.

In *Trust the Wings*, her debut novel, Barbara fictionalizes many of her unforgettable experiences to reveal the unpredictable challenges for all caregivers and home care professionals. But she also illuminates the personally satisfying successes and the joys of home care and affirms those who are called by work or life to serve others in times of need.